Acclaim for Michael Korda's

MAN TO MAN

"Bravo to the courageous Mr. Korda. . . . A writer of great skill, Korda grips the reader with a step-by-step, unblinking account of his own personal battle. . . . Husbands and wives who read this book together will come away strengthened by its message." —Gail Sheehy

"Michael Korda has performed a medical public service. . . . I was stunned by his candor and moved by his courage."

—Dominick Dunne

"The best book about prostate surgery that I have ever read. . . . Korda brilliantly takes you through the whole process in a very worthwhile read." —Larry King, *USA Today*

"Necessarily frank and undeniably fascinating. . . . Extremely valuable for its blunt candor, no-nonsense advice and message of survival."

—*Seattle Times*

"A book for all men who are in or are approaching their 'prostate years,' an unflinching guide. . . . Korda knows how to put his message across in a rip-snorting, page-turning narrative style."

—*Cleveland Plain Dealer*

Michael Korda

MAN TO MAN

Michael Korda is the editor-in-chief of Simon & Schuster as well as the author of an acclaimed book about his family, *Charmed Lives*; several successful novels; and the number-one bestseller *Power*. He lives with his wife, Margaret, in Dutchess County, New York.

MAN TO MAN

MICHAEL KORDA

MAN TO MAN

SURVIVING PROSTATE CANCER

VINTAGE BOOKS

A Division of Random House, Inc.

New York

The Library of Congress has cataloged the Random House edition as follows:
Korda, Michael.
Man to man: surviving prostate cancer / Michael Korda.
p. cm.
Includes bibliographical references.
ISBN 0-679-44844-6
1. Korda, Michael.—Health.
2. Prostate—Cancer—Patients—United States—Biography.
I. Title.
RC280.P7K67 1996
362.1'9699463—dc20
[B] 95-53314

Vintage ISBN: 0-679-78123-4

Book design by Tanya M. Pérez-Rock

Random House Web address: http://www.randomhouse.com/

Printed in the United States of America
10 9 8 7 6 5 4 3 2 1

FOR MARGARET

Without whom . . .

ACKNOWLEDGMENTS

I am completely responsible for any errors in this book, but I would like to thank Avodah Offit, M.D., and Lenard Jacobson, M.D., for their careful reading and correction of the manuscript.

I owe far too much to far too many people to list them all, but I would particularly like to single out Dennis O'Hara, the organizer of the Poughkeepsie prostate-cancer group; Rebecca Head, for her unfailing support over more years than either of us would care to admit; Chuck Adams, for taking on his shoulders the burden of my work during my recuperation; Richard and Roxanne Bacon, Dot Burnett, and Emory Smith, who did so much to help my recovery; Cher, for her unfailingly positive long-distance support; Larry McMurtry, for always being there despite problems of his own; Rod Barker and Peter Forbath, for friendship above and beyond the call of duty; and Carol Bowie, for her unflagging retyping of the manuscript.

CONTENTS

PART ONE

THE SILENT KILLER

1

EVERY YEAR MORE THAN 200,000 AMERICAN MEN ARE TOLD THEY have prostate cancer. Nearly 50,000 of them die, many of them needlessly.

Prostate cancer is the male equivalent of breast cancer—the numbers are almost identical—though it receives considerably less attention. Fashion models are photographed wearing designer T-shirts with a target printed over their breasts to remind the public about the dangers of breast cancer, but there is no equivalent campaign for men. Few black-tie dinners or theater benefits are given in aid of prostate-cancer research. Rather like the prostate itself, prostate cancer remains stubbornly invisible.

It resembles breast cancer in ways that go beyond the merely statistical. Just as breast cancer is the biggest fear of most women—formerly unspoken, but no longer—prostate cancer is the biggest fear of most men. It carries with it not only the fear of dying, like all cancer, but fears that go to the very core of masculinity—for the treatment of prostate cancer, whatever form it takes, almost invariably carries with it well-known risks of incontinence and impotence that strike directly at any man's self-image, pride, and enjoyment of life, and which, by their very nature, tend to make men reticent on the subject.

It is precisely this reticence which makes prostate cancer such a deadly, silent scourge. Women talk to each other about their bodies; men do not—still less so when their ability to function sexually is at risk.

As a result, men who have prostate cancer all too often feel themselves isolated at the very first mention of the bad news, unable to share their worst fears with anybody. To the fear, which is perfectly natural, of death, loss of virility, and incontinence is therefore added a dreadful loneliness; for unlike women, who tend to bond together in distress, men—certainly in the face of *this* disease—tend to retreat into silence. For many of them, prostate cancer is a *private* battle, and because of that, it is all too often lost.

THIS BOOK IS an attempt to break through that barrier of silence and isolation to write about prostate cancer—about *surviving* it successfully—with a frankness that I myself have found lacking in every book on the subject, and to make the experience less fearful by being truthful about it. I mean this book to be hopeful—the key word is *survival.* I also mean it to be realistic.

It is, of course, only one man's story, but I have talked to many other survivors of prostate cancer, as well as to doctors, nurses, and therapists, so it is also the story of many other people. Of course, every case of cancer is as individual as the person whose life it threatens; still, everybody who has had prostate cancer shares certain fears, experiences, and doubts: it is a kind of community, with its own language, its own key questions ("What was your PSA* level?";

---

* PSA stands for Prostate Specific Antigen, and is used here to signify the blood test that is commonly used to determine whether a patient may be at risk for prostate cancer.

"Did they get it all out?"; "When did you regain continence?"; "Have you had an erection yet?"), its own lore, its own heroes and villains.

Membership is simple, and not dependent on race, creed, religion, or sexual preference (though gender here matters—this is still an all-male club and certain to remain so, perhaps the last one): all you have to do to join is be told by your doctor after your next annual physical examination that you have a suspiciously high PSA level, or an irregularity on the prostate during the course of what ought to be your doctor's annual digital rectal examination (DRE) of that organ, followed by a positive biopsy (about which more later), and you're in, no questions asked, welcome to the club.

—∾—

I JOINED THE club, unexpectedly, in the autumn of 1994—it was a Thursday in October, at about two-thirty in the afternoon.

A few days before, my internist had called me after my annual physical examination to say that my PSA level had risen from 15 the year before to 22.

I wasn't unduly alarmed, nor did he seem to be. A biopsy done the previous year had proved negative for cancer. I did not think I had anything to worry about.

Some people, I had been assured at the time, particularly those like myself with an enlarged prostate, tend to run high PSA levels without cancer. All the same, another biopsy was indicated, so, since my own urologist was away, I made an appointment at the Prostate Cancer Detection Center of Memorial Sloan-Kettering Hospital, in New York City, which specializes in cancer, and had it done, much as I disliked the procedure. I felt good about being cautious and taking sensible precautions, but in no way anxious.

I phoned Kathy, a cheerful young nurse at the Prostate Cancer Detection Center, for the results of my biopsy before I went to lunch, but we failed to make contact, so I left a message. I returned from lunch, took off my coat, and sat down to call her again, when the phone rang and I picked it up. It was Kathy, calling me.

My mind was on the work that lay before me on my desk—calls to make, people to see, the usual overload of book publishing. "Hi," I said. "Sorry we missed each other this morning."

"That's okay," she said. "I have your results."

"Great," I said. She had a nice voice, I thought. Upbeat, all-American, perky, even a little sexy in a lively, wholesome way; the kind of voice I associate with cheerleaders and homecoming queens and the Midwest.

There was a pause, a hesitation long enough for me to wonder if she'd been interrupted. Then she said one word, "Unfortunately," and I guessed what was coming next.

Unfortunately. The word echoed in my mind as she talked to me. Unfortunately, the results of the biopsy were positive. Unfortunately, I would need to schedule a CAT scan, an MRI, a bone scan, and X rays as soon as possible to determine whether or not the cancer had spread—the sooner the better, Kathy made it clear. Dr. Russo would see me—*and my wife,* she emphasized—the next week to review the findings of these tests and discuss treatment. She read off a list of names and phone numbers. Did I have any questions?

I had none, except for a foolish desire to ask Kathy if she did, indeed, come from the Midwest. I wrote down all the information numbly, as if none of it had anything to do with me. "I have cancer," I said to myself silently, but I wasn't sure I believed it yet, and already guessed how much harder it would be to say it out loud.

Kathy and I said good-bye to each other—how many times a day does she break this news, I wondered, and how does she manage to be so pleasant while doing it?—then I sat for a few moments staring at the piece of paper before me, with the scribbled names and numbers of physicians whose skills I had never dreamed of needing, and on whom my life now, apparently, depended.

Nothing, I thought, would be the same from now on.

—m—

I PICKED UP the telephone and dialed my wife, Margaret, in the country. "I got my results," I said, striving too hard for a neutral tone.

"And?"

I hesitated and took the plunge. "They were positive."

"What does that mean?" I could hear fear in her voice, like an electric current between us. People who have been married long enough hear feelings in each other's voices, even in their silences.

"I have cancer." There. For the first time, I had said aloud the phrase that would soon become familiar when talking to friends or with doctors, technicians, and nurses. *I have cancer.* Very soon I would be able to speak those words without feeling self-conscious about them, as if they represented a perfectly ordinary statement of fact. For the moment, they created a kind of dead, heavy silence, which neither one of us seemed eager to break.

Until a few minutes ago, I reflected, I had assumed myself to be a reasonably healthy man—with some pride, I should add, for I had given up smoking six years earlier, I ate and drank moderately, and I ran, worked out at the gym, or swam every day. Now I had cancer. You can't, I thought, get more unhealthy than *that.* It didn't seem fair. I reminded myself that Jack Kennedy was fond of pointing out *life* isn't fair, but it didn't help much. It didn't help *him* much, either, in the end.

"How do you feel?" Margaret's voice was trembling slightly, as if she were on the verge of tears. I wished I were home, instead of ninety miles away, in the city. I would rather have held her when I told her the news—and been held, for that matter—but she knew I was expecting the results.

"I feel okay," I said cautiously. "No different than I did before the news. I guess that will change."

It wasn't so, though—I *did* feel different. I sensed that I had crossed some invisible line into a new phase of my life, the way a traveler might feel when crossing a frontier and entering a different country, with a strange language, new customs, different rules, signs that made no sense, policemen with unfamiliar uniforms pacing in pairs up and down the railway platforms. I was entering—had already entered—the country of the seriously ill, and no doubt I would soon have to learn its customs, its language, its rules. Until a few minutes ago I could have said about any catastrophe "Well, at least I've still got my health" or "At least I don't have cancer." I no longer had my health; I *did* have cancer. The unspoken worst fear had come true. I would never have to be afraid of having cancer again. I had it. I told that to Margaret.

She thought about it, and concluded, I suspect, that I was being too calm for my own good. "You'd better come home right away," she said.

But I couldn't. She had gone back to the country—we live about ninety miles north of New York City, in Dutchess County—with the car on Tuesday. I was being picked up by a hired car at five. I explained all this, as if any of it mattered by comparison with the bad news.

"How bad is it going to be?" Margaret asked with a depth of concern I had never heard before.

"Lots of people survive prostate cancer," I said, striving for a confident tone. "It's slow-growing. There are a lot of things they can do."

I said this to cheer her up. The truth was that while I didn't know much about it, prostate cancer scared the shit out of me. The only two people I knew closely who had it, died of it, descending by small, agonizing steps into a world of such pain and suffering that those who loved them prayed only for their death. Cornelius Ryan, the author of *The Longest Day*, had not only died that way but had written a harrowing book about his struggle with prostate cancer, which I had edited and published, and which haunted me for years. I had also worked with Leo Szilard, the great Hungarian physicist, on his last book, *The Voice of the Dolphins*, and visited him almost daily at Memorial Hospital as he fought to finish it before death took him, bloated, pasty-faced, in agony. As a result, ironically, cancer of the prostate was one of my nightmare fears, the disease I knew best and feared most.

As if those two exposures to prostate cancer weren't enough, two people I knew had just died of it—Steve Ross, the CEO of Time-Warner, and Anatole Broyard, the *New York Times* book critic. In both their cases, the disease had been quite the reverse of slow-growing, and nothing the doctors could do had helped much.

"It's strange," I said. "In retrospect, I should have *known*. When Russo and Fleishner, the doctors at the Prostate Cancer Detection Center, were looking at the ultrasound picture of my prostate, they kept exchanging glances, as if they were saying, 'Uh-oh, do you see what I see?' And when I told Dr. Russo I had really *hated* having the biopsy done last year, he put his hand on my shoulder, remember?, and told me, 'If you were my own *brother*, I would urge you to have this done right now.' "

That was the point, I now realized, at which I should have been scared shitless. Russo had spoken with such vehemence that I had been taken aback. After all, there he was, a total stranger, his hand gripping my shoulder, talking to me as if I really *were* his brother, his face close to mine, his dark eyes full of emotion, not at all one's picture of the cold, detached surgeon.

"I've had a bad feeling about this from the beginning," Margaret said.

I was surprised. I hadn't. It's not that I'm an incorrigible optimist, either—on the contrary, I usually expect the worst—but somehow I had managed to armor myself against the possibility of *any* serious disease striking me, let alone cancer, irrationally convinced that it wasn't going to happen to *me*. Nothing short of Kathy's flat statement of fact, however pleasantly delivered, would have been likely to breach my defenses. Margaret's intuition, as usual, had been correct.

"Don't worry," I said as firmly as I could, conscious that I was whistling in the dark. "Everything's going to be fine."

We hung up and I stared out the window at a bright autumn afternoon. I had not convinced Margaret for a moment that everything was going to be fine.

As a matter of fact, I didn't believe a word of it myself.

—⁓—

I'M AN EDITOR and a writer. Faced with any problem, the first thing I want to do is read about it. I went downstairs to one of the big bookstores in Rockefeller Center and browsed glumly through the Health/Medicine section. I felt an irrational resentment against people who were looking for lighter reading, together with a slight, if inappropriate, sense of shame, like somebody furtively glancing at the XXX-rated tapes in a video store.

At first sight, there didn't seem much to choose from—there were dozens of books on breast cancer, but hardly any on the prostate. The few there were, were way down on the very bottom shelf, so that I had to get down on my knees with my head tilted sideways close to the floor to peer at the titles through the reading part of my glasses.

I could find only two books—one a jaunty personal memoir called *My Prostate and Me,* by William Martin, with a smiling photograph of the author on the cover, looking healthy and, presumably, cured; the other a somewhat more daunting volume by Stephen N. Rous, M.D., called *The Prostate Book.* I also picked out a fat paperback, *Choices: Realistic Alternatives in Cancer Treatment,* written by Marion Morra and Eve Potts, and mostly in question-and-answer form. I skipped through it as I was waiting in line to pay, my eye stopping sharply on a question in boldface type near the end of the book: "**How can the patient be helped to die in comfort?**"

There was a pretty girl behind the cash register who might have given me a flirtatious smile if I'd handed over three racy novels—it was the middle of the afternoon, and there weren't many customers to keep her busy—but one glance at the titles of my purchases and her face turned to stone as she rang them up. She managed to take my credit card without eye contact. She handed me my package.

"Thanks," I said, but she was already looking toward the next cus-tomer as if I didn't exist. My choice of books clearly marked me as somebody bearing bad news, either my own or somebody else's. We all know how people feel about messengers bearing bad news.

I went back to the office and spent the rest of the afternoon telling the news to those few friends and close colleagues who I thought ab-solutely had to know. One of my closest friends, a CEO, warned me, when it was already too late, not to tell anyone at work. "You'll see," he said. "They'll write you off. Don't say I didn't warn you."

That thought had not crossed my mind, but once he had put it there it stayed, depressing me even further. This, as I was to discover, is in fact a serious problem for a lot of men. Cancer can spell the end of a career, on top of all its other horrors. On the one hand, you can't keep it secret in the long run from the people you work for; on the other hand, they may decide that a man with prostate cancer is a bad risk.

As with many of the dilemmas that confront the man with prostate cancer, there is no easy solution to this one. My own was to tell the truth to anyone who would listen. You need all the help you can get. Other people's sympathy and support count for a lot, and you're not going to get that if you keep the fact that you have cancer a secret—which you can't do forever anyway.

By the time I'd broken the news to perhaps half a dozen people, I was exhausted, both by their emotions and my own. Once I was in the car, I was tempted to sleep, but decided not to put off my reading.

If I had been under any illusion about the gravity of the news, Dr. Rous's book would have dispelled it. Rous, a distinguished urologist, did not pull his punches—the words *incontinence, impotence,* and *death* seemed to proliferate in the text and the index, though they were overshadowed by the illustrations, reproduced in sharp detail and remarkably high quality. I carefully studied an X ray of a skele-ton showing "a strongly positive bone scan . . . due to an extensive spread of cancer of the prostate," then moved on, with a rapidly sink-ing heart, to pictures of biopsy needles, an artificial urinary sphincter, and penile prostheses. The full weight of the word *spread*—as in "spread beyond the prostate" or "spread to the bone"—dawned on me, as did the importance of the tests Kathy had urged me to schedule as soon as possible.

I had not, until now, given serious thought to the subject of death, but Dr. Rous brought it home to me, with cool, clinical understatement, as the car took me home. I stared out at the autumn foliage, at its blazing peak. It occurred to me that I might not be around to see it the next year. I took a certain wry satisfaction from the coincidence that Margaret and I had only just signed our new wills after months of meetings with our lawyer and our financial adviser.

I wondered whether our signing them had, in fact, been a grim coincidence. During the whole interminable process, the cancer had been inside me, growing silently all the time. Had my subconscious known it was there? Was that the reason I had pushed Margaret, always reluctant to involve herself in legal and financial matters, to come into the city and attend the meetings?

I tried to think if there had been *any* signs of cancer that I'd ignored or repressed, but on the spur of the moment I could think of nothing significant, unless it was a certain amount of fatigue over the past year or so, a feeling that I tired more easily than in the past and needed more rest.

That, as I was to discover, is perhaps the most sinister fact about prostate cancer: in most cases there *are* no warning symptoms—no pain, no discomfort, nothing that would sound an alarm to even the most careful of hypochondriacs. Prostate cancer creeps up on its victim silently, often striking men who appear to be 100 percent fit and healthy, like me. The words most often heard by urologists on informing a patient that he has prostate cancer are "But I've never felt better in my life," and alas, it is mostly true.

I skipped to the end of Dr. Rous's book—I would read it with considerably more attention later—and decided that I didn't want to know about further complications of prostate surgery just at the moment. After all, as yet I didn't even know if surgery was called for. It might not be necessary, I told myself optimistically: Dr. Rous's book had sections on radiation, hormone treatments, and "watchful wait-ing"—essentially, doing nothing and keeping an eye on the PSA at regular intervals—which had a definite appeal. Then it dawned on me that worse than surgery itself would be the possibility that it was already too late for surgery. I picked up William Martin's book.

My Prostate and Me, which bore quotes on the back of the dust jacket from Jerry Lewis and Senator Robert Dole, quickly had me feeling more cheerful. Unlike Dr. Rous, whose knowledge of the prostate was both complete and apocalyptic, Martin, a professor of sociology at Rice University in Houston, Texas, presented the reader only with his own experience as a patient who had undergone a rad-ical prostatectomy for prostate cancer. His tone—and message—were distinctly upbeat and reassuring. Like me, he had been shocked and horrified to learn that he had cancer, but his surgery had been successful, he admired and liked his surgeon, and his recovery had been swift and painless.

I was delighted to read not only Professor Martin's report that he had recovered full continence within two or three days of the re-moval of his Foley catheter (about which more later, I'm afraid), but his confession, expressed with a certain elephantine shyness, that he had been able to show his wife an erection only nine days after the re-moval of his prostate (he placed her hand on the organ, an event, he noted with touching accuracy, that occurred at exactly "6:41 A.M. on November 24, 1993"). Sex between them had resumed ("budded," to use his exact word) less than six weeks after the operation.

Professor Martin did not devote a lot of space to his stay in the hospital, but since his only complaint was that the nurses were slow in responding to calls—a complaint so universal as to be meaning-less—it didn't sound too bad. His conclusion about his experience with prostate cancer was that it was "one of the richest episodes of [his] life."

I was doubtful that I would find it one of the richest episodes of mine; still, I felt a lot better about things by the time I put his book down with the fading of the light and closed my eyes. Surgery scared me almost as much as death itself—maybe more, since death seemed abstract, whereas surgery was something I could imagine all too clearly, with a sharp, hard-edged precision derived, no doubt, from countless movies and television series: the rows of cold, gleaming instruments, the glaring lights, the splashes of blood—*my* blood—against the pale blue or green of the surgeons' disposable gowns. . . . Somewhere in Dr. Rous's book he made a point of the fact that a radical prostatectomy was a serious business, *major* surgery.

When a *surgeon* gives you a warning that a procedure is *"major,"* watch out, I thought.

———— ✦ ————

IT WAS LATE when I arrived home. I dragged my shopping bags full of manuscripts—the backbreaking burden of every book editor—into the house. Margaret embraced me, and I made us a drink.

Incongruous as it had seemed in my office that I had cancer, it seemed even more so at home. I felt no different, nor was there any difference in the small rituals (who doesn't have them?) of my arrival home at the end of a busy week. I had brought food up from the city from my weekly early-morning shopping trip to Zabar's, the famous delicatessen on Broadway. We fussed amicably, as we always do, over what goes where in the refrigerator and freezer. It was as if the two of us were locked firmly on autopilot, clinging to our usual routines as if for dear life.

"Cheers," I said. We clinked our glasses. The sound did not cheer either of us. "I've been reading up on prostate cancer," I told Margaret.

"Is that wise? Why not wait until you've had the tests and seen the doctor? Reading about it is just going to make you depressed. Or frightened."

"No, no, it's had just the opposite effect." It was true. Information comforts me. I like to *know* things. "Anyway," I went on, "I'm not trying to turn myself into a doctor overnight or anything like that. If

I don't know anything about prostate cancer, how am I even going to know what questions to ask?"

"I would have thought that the only question worth asking is 'Am I going to get better?'" Margaret hadn't touched her drink. "I can't believe we're having this conversation," she said. "Yesterday we were talking about going to Santa Fe for Thanksgiving and Christmas, and today we're talking about cancer."

"I brought up a list of dates and flights in my briefcase," I said. We usually spend a couple of weeks in Santa Fe during the winter. I love it there, and think of it as my second home, but it suddenly seemed remote, far away, hardly even *real,* like the far side of the moon. Whatever our plans were going to be for the coming winter, I did not think they would include Santa Fe. Would I ever see it again? I wondered. The question was macabre, but not entirely unrealistic. "Somehow, I don't think we'll be going there for a while."

Margaret's eyes looked bruised. She wasn't crying, but it occurred to me that she had had the whole afternoon to cry. It might have been kinder to have broken the news when I got home, but it was too late now. "This is going to take over our lives, isn't it?" she asked sadly.

She was right, of course. I could already see how cancer would come to dominate our lives, as it had dominated the lives of many people we knew. For a time—sometimes a long time, sometimes even for what remained of their lives—cancer became the only thing they could think about; all their energies were spent in fighting it. Nothing outside their struggle to survive existed until the cancer finally won, or was beaten back into remission, a kind of uneasy truce.

I made a mental note that I must not let this happen to us, that it was conceding a kind of victory by default to cancer. It was a resolution that I would not be able to keep. "It may, for a while," I said cautiously. "We must try not to let it."

Margaret looked skeptical—correctly, as it turned out. "What do we do now?" she asked.

"We wait. We wait until next week, for more tests. Then we wait until Dr. Russo has studied the results. Then he'll tell us what he thinks. Kathy says he'll give us all the time we want to ask him questions." Since at first glance Dr. Russo gave off the unmistakable impression of a man for whom every second counted (it takes one to know one), that, as much as anything else his nurse had to say, had made me realize the gravity of the news.

"Tell me about the tests."

Resisting the temptation to display my newfound knowledge, I told her the gist of what I had gleaned from reading the two books—briefly, that if the results were positive, that is, if cancer had spread to the bone or other organs, the future was grim, altogether eclipsing today's bad news.

"You mean, on top of bad news there could be worse news?"

"Much worse."

We were silent for a moment.

"You're very calm about it," Margaret said.

"Not really. I'm just too scared to show it, probably. It's not so hard to be calm about this part of it—bad news probably produces an adrenaline rush, like being in an accident or getting shot. Besides, I don't know the worst of it yet. Even then, it isn't knowing I *have* cancer that frightens me. What frightens me is what's to come—the operation, or the radiation treatments, or the chemo, or whatever, all the things I hoped would never happen to me. Pain—*that's* what's scary. And death, of course."

"You're not going to die."

"It does happen."

"It's not going to happen to you."

Margaret spoke with such conviction that I almost believed her. If she had decided she wasn't going to let me die, who was I to argue with her? After all, like most beautiful women, she usually got her way.

"Why don't you take a tranquilizer?" she asked.

"It won't change anything. And I'm not untranquil."

"Then let's finish our drinks, have our dinner, watch *ER,* and go to bed," she said, and that's what we did. When in doubt, do what you would normally do—that had always been our way of meeting a crisis, and there are worse ways.

We fell asleep that night in each other's arms, and had never felt closer.

In the middle of the night, with the moonlight streaming in and Margaret beside me, it seemed hard to believe that something inside me was trying its damnedest to kill me. I shut my eyes and tried to sleep again. I felt as if there were a stranger in the bed with us. The stranger, of course, was cancer.

That was the first day of my illness—of *knowing* about it, anyway.

2

HOW LONG I'D HAD IT *WITHOUT* KNOWING ABOUT IT IS ANYBODY'S guess. Prostate cancer is notoriously slow-growing, but it can also move with the swiftness of a prairie fire, and with much the same devastating effect. In my case, it also was masked by the fact that I'd had "prostate troubles" for years.

Lots of men ignore their prostate, hardly even know where it *is,* until it suddenly claims their full attention when they are diagnosed with cancer. My prostate and I, however, were already on familiar, if uncordial, terms.

For a couple of years before my sixtieth birthday, my prostate had been making its presence felt in my life, at first in small, uncomfortable ways, then more persistently.

At the beginning, I did not take it seriously—the prostate is one of the few organs that lends itself to humor, at any rate of the Borscht Belt type, and the symptoms of an enlarging prostate are the subject of many coarse jokes and comedians' shticks: after all, difficulty in urination is one of the better-known humiliations of the aging process in men. Who does not have some member of the family who has to get up several times a night, who can't pee when he wants to, or can't *stop* from peeing just when it's most inconvenient (an automobile trip, for instance), or who can't seem to get rid of the last drop of urine before he zips up his fly, leaving an embarrassing dark spot on his trousers? "Old age," Charles de Gaulle wrote in his war memoirs, "is a shipwreck," but before the ship goes down there is usually time to experience a lot of small humiliations, many of them centered on the prostate.

If an enlarged prostate is common among older men, that does not mean it is *confined* to the elderly—not all. Many men in their forties, even more in their fifties, experience the symptoms of what doctors refer to as "benign prostatic hyperplasia," or BPH, a sure sign of which is the attention they find themselves paying to those road signs on the interstate highways which indicate the distance to the next comfort station, or the fact that the first thing they do on entering any public building is to take note of where the men's room is.

In my case, at the beginning, the problem came and went unpredictably. For long periods, I was fine. Then, out of the blue, I would find myself plotting my course through midtown Manhattan to take advantage of the men's rooms in hotel lobbies or department stores on my flight path. I learned where the men's room was hidden away in Saks Fifth Avenue, in the underground concourse of Rockefeller Center, in the Waldorf-Astoria Hotel, at the Donnell Library on Fifty-third Street—for most public toilets are hard to find and obscurely sign-posted, no doubt to protect them from being used by casual strangers off the street. Some shops, I discovered, will let you use the employees' toilet if you spend enough money.

Commuting back and forth between the city and our home in Dutchess County made me an expert in the availability (and cleanliness) of men's rooms in gas stations and motels along the Sawmill, Hutchinson, and Taconic parkways. I developed a small fetish for preempting an aisle seat at the movies so that I could get up and go to the bathroom without having to bother people.

The symptoms would appear, go on for a while, then disappear as mysteriously as they had come. At first, I assumed they were from a bladder infection. My doctor suggested I take Urised, which acts as a sedative to the bladder, and I soon became a Urised junkie, especially after I discovered that you didn't need a new prescription to get more. It *did* appear to cut down the frequency and urgency of urination a little, though at the price of turning my urine a bright purple.

I went on like this for a couple of years—the problem did not seem like a major one; it was intermittent, with long spells between attacks; and when it happened, the medication helped. It did not seem like anything worth worrying about—although, subtly, without even noticing, I had in fact begun to alter my life in small ways, like planning my driving around known rest stops.

Then, during an annual physical examination, after having given me the usual digital rectal examination—an experience I have always loathed—my internist commented on the fact that my prostate seemed "a little boggy."

Boggy? It seemed an odd word to apply to an organ. I asked him what he meant. He shrugged. It was a bit enlarged, he said, and soft. I might have an infection of the prostate—prostatitis, it was called. Nothing to worry about, but it would probably do no harm to see a urologist. I resisted the idea. Everything I knew about urology told me I wouldn't like the experience a bit. Couldn't I just take an antibiotic? Sure, he said, and wrote me a prescription for one. But just as a precaution, he added, I ought to see a specialist anyway.

I put it off—put it out of mind, actually. The problem cleared up for a while, maybe because of the antibiotic, maybe of its own volition.

A few months later, without warning, driving down to the city late one winter night when all the gas stations were closed and their bathrooms locked, a normal commute turned into a nightmare journey. A sudden, intense urge to urinate, beginning suddenly, appearing, as it were, out of nowhere, had me parking my car illegally every ten or fifteen minutes or so on the shoulder of the road so I could climb over frozen snowbanks in my loafers to pee in the shelter of the woods, only to have to do it all over again a few miles farther along. When I got to the West Side Highway, I had to pull over and urinate on the spot—I couldn't wait another second—at a point where there's a space for police and emergency vehicles just south of 125th Street. Traffic streamed by. Everybody, I felt sure, was staring at me as I tried ineffectively to conceal what I was doing behind the door of my car. Would the police come along? I wondered. Was it not a misdemeanor to urinate in public? Homeless people and drunks did it all the time in New York City, of course, and got away with it, but surely I was expected to know better and would be treated more harshly.

I felt a confused mixture of shame, guilt, and fear at my loss of control, coupled with inexpressible physical relief as I emptied my bladder in full sight of the world. Less than a quarter of an hour later, however, when I got to my garage, I had to leave in the car my shopping bags full of work and make a mad dash for the service elevator, praying that it wasn't in use. I danced from one foot to the other in agony all the way up to the fifty-third floor, desperate not to wet my pants—or the elevator floor. I was already unzipping myself with one hand while I was unlocking the door of my apartment with the other, and only just made it in time. It seemed hard to believe that the human body could contain so much liquid, or that trying to hold it back could be so painful.

There was no putting the matter off any longer. In the morning, I made an appointment with the urologist recommended by my doctor, and found myself in his waiting room the next day with a fair number of middle-aged men—"suits," as young people now call middle-aged executives—most of them looking slightly ashamed of themselves, as if merely being there was an indication of problems they wanted to hide. All of us, I noticed, looked around to make sure where the toilet was. And most of us got up to use it at least once while waiting to see the doctor.

I was finally shown into the urologist's handsome, wood-paneled office. He was a tweed-clad, stern-looking man in his late fifties who listened to the story of my woes without expression, as if he had heard it a thousand times before—as was surely the case. "Let's have a look at you," he said, and led me next door into an examination room, where I bent over in what was soon to become a familiar posture while he performed a brisk digital probe of my prostate.

"It's enlarged, all right," he said.

"Boggy, would you say?"

He raised an eyebrow, annoyed, I assumed, with the imprecision of the word *boggy*. It was on the tip of my tongue to point out that it was my internist's description, not mine, but I decided not to. "The prostate is *enlarged*," he repeated with emphasis. "It's common enough in men your age. Nothing to worry about."

"I see. What can be done about it, though? I'm taking an antibiotic."

He shrugged. "There might be some infection," he said, though he didn't seem much concerned about the possibility. "Leave a urine sample for my nurse. Keep taking the antibiotic. Drink plenty of fluids. Cranberry juice is good. Ejaculation helps. You get rid of the prostatic fluids that way. Have plenty of sex, that's my advice. The more, the better. If necessary, masturbate. Call me in a couple of weeks."

I laughed. "My God, if *that's* all it takes . . ." I pulled up my trousers. I was wondering if I had conveyed to him just how severe my discomfort was—I have a tendency not to paint too dark a picture when talking to doctors, a residue of stoicism and reserve that comes, no doubt, from an English education and from not wanting to be thought a sissy or a whiner. "I'm not sure if I've made it clear just how hard all this peeing is to take, doctor," I said. "Once I get into one of these cycles, it never stops. The moment I've urinated, I want to start urinating again. . . ." The doctor nodded impatiently, his hand on the doorknob—either I was telling him something he already knew, which was very likely, or, having given me his diagnosis, he felt that he was through with me. I wondered if I had *overdone* it, perhaps—if he felt that I was a hypochondriac, wasting his time with small complaints when he had patients with more serious problems to see. I tried for the lighter touch. "I'm beginning to feel I could write a guide to the men's rooms of New York."

He did not smile. "Some change in the pattern of urination is normal at a certain age," he said as he went out the door. "Good afternoon."

I felt foolish, as if I had indeed wasted his time. If cranberry juice and sex were all it took to cure me, then my problem could surely not be serious. I began a regime of both as quickly as I could, while continuing with the antibiotic and the Urised, and within a few days my urinary timetable resumed its normal pattern, I was able to drive home without incident, I slept through the night without having to get up, and I no longer needed to hang around the rest rooms of midtown Manhattan and Westchester and Putnam counties like some kind of guilty pervert.

The urologist might be short on human warmth and bedside manner, but I was grateful all the same, though not eager to see him again.

—⁂—

SLOWLY, HOWEVER, MY enlarged prostate began to make its presence felt in my life. Whereas in the early days of my experience with BPH the most obvious symptom of distress had been frequent urination, now, unpredictably, I would find that I couldn't urinate when I wanted to, or only with great difficulty, as the urine slowed to an unsteady trickle. The prostate was sensitive, too. Most of my adult life I've enjoyed riding. Soon I found that I needed a sheepskin pad on the saddle to cushion my crotch, then a foam pillow. Finally it became apparent that whatever I did, riding aggravated my prostate troubles, and I found myself taking shorter rides, then avoiding trotting or jumping, then riding less frequently, and finally not riding at all.

Things got worse. I invested in a "rubber doughnut," which I took with me to the movies and to restaurants and kept on the driver's seat of my car. I was not becoming an invalid, by any stretch of the imagination, but gradually, small step by small step, I was slipping into an invalid life, no longer doing what *I* wanted to do but what my prostate allowed me to.

In a small way—a very small way, compared to what was to come—my prostate troubles brought me face-to-face with the concept of "quality of life" (a phrase much in vogue among doctors) for the first time, and I didn't like it a bit. Things I used to do with ease, I no longer could, and while they weren't necessarily *important* things, the process filled me with foreboding. Already, my prostate was beginning to affect my sex life, despite the urologist's prescription to have as much sex as possible.

The prostate lies in intimate connection with the male sexual organs, and plays a by-no-means-modest role in male sexuality. When the prostate is of normal size, healthy, and doing its humdrum job, it goes unnoticed. Once it becomes enlarged, sick, or balky, it quickly makes its presence known.

Most men with BPH seem to experience some waning of sexuality, a nagging sense that something is no longer as it should be, as if the malaise of the prostate is spreading. Probably it is nothing more than the fact that any discomfort, infection, or swelling in one organ is likely to have an effect on the others it is connected to; still, there it is—prostate trouble is almost always accompanied by sexual difficulties, partly out of a self-fulfilling fear, partly because it tends to focus the mind, when it comes to that area of the body, on the problems of urination to the exclusion of anything else. A man who can't stop urinating—or, perhaps worse, can't *start*—is unlikely to be in the mood for love—or, for that matter, to make much headway as an object of romance.

Nor is he likely to receive much in the way of sympathy from the woman in his life. Women have their own problems in this territory, particularly those who have had children, and in any case they don't share all those old-fashioned male myths, celebrated in barrooms, boarding schools, locker rooms, and the armed services, that center around being able to knock back beer after beer without having to go to the bathroom, or pissing with a strong, steady stream.

In the postfeminist world women may *use* the phrase "pissing contest," but only men can actually *engage* in one, or can at least remember doing so as boys. Boys compete to see who can piss the farthest, as they do to see who can ejaculate the farthest—a lot of male mythology's central core of belief is centered on just those abilities that an enlarged prostate compromises, which makes it, for most men, a singularly depressing condition, not dramatic enough to attract pity, but in some way undermining many of the more cherished masculine attributes. It is hardly surprising that so many men simply hide their condition, from their wives, from their doctors, even—and perhaps most of all—from themselves.

Certainly I did my best to ignore my problem, or hide it, and became quite an expert at slipping out of meetings, ostensibly to take a telephone call, when, in fact, I was on my way to the bathroom. I knew I was going to have to see the urologist again, and I put it off every day. In the end, it was something that happened to my friend Arthur that finally drove me back to the urologist.

Arthur, a fellow about my age, was, it turned out, another secret sufferer from BPH; his knowledge of the men's rooms on the roads between the East Side and Connecticut was as encyclopedic as mine was of midtown Manhattan and the parkways to upstate New York.

Naturally, I hadn't known that Arthur was a fellow sufferer. Being men, neither of us had revealed his condition to the other. Arthur, however, had the misfortune one day to take an over-the-counter cold medicine without reading the microscopic note on the label warning men with prostate problems not to use it, and shortly thereafter found himself being rushed to the hospital with complete urinary blockage. He was reticent, in his gentlemanly way, about the operation and its consequences, but confided in an unguarded moment that he now ejaculated backward into his bladder ("retrograde ejaculation" is the exact medical phrase), a notion that I found hard to imagine, and he impossible to describe.

POOR ARTHUR'S CASE was vividly in my mind when I finally returned to my urologist. Once again he performed a DRE (I was already beginning to hate the crisp sound of the surgical glove snapping as he put it on), and once again we went back to his book-lined office after I had cleaned myself off and pulled my trousers back up.

My prostate was somewhat more enlarged than before, he said—nothing to worry about, but it would certainly explain the symptoms about which I was complaining.

There was a long silence. Was there anything to be done about this? I asked. Surgery was one option, he said, making a steeple of his fingers. I must think of the prostate as shaped like an apple, he explained. He mimed an apple with his hands. The urethra ran through what might be thought of as the core of the apple. When the prostate became enlarged, the urethra was compressed, and the flow of urine thereby slowed. As a result, the bladder had to work harder to push the urine through the narrowed passage, and this led to the thickening of the wall of the bladder, which, like any muscle, built itself up the more it was exercised, creating more problems.

Surgery, he went on, was the best solution, the "gold standard" against which all other therapies were measured.

What *kind* of surgery? I asked. He was more cheerful now that we were on the subject of surgery. Urology is a surgical specialty. Urologists are therefore all surgeons, men of action, true believers in their own skill and the technology at their command; the prospect of solving the patient's problems with a scalpel generally appeals to them a lot more than sitting around talking to the patient. There were several approaches, he said, warming to his subject, all of which involved removing enough tissue to free the pressure on the urethra and open up a strong, steady flow of urine. My quality of life, he assured me, would improve immediately. One possibility—perhaps the most popular—was a transurethral resection of the prostate (referred to as a TURP), in which an instrument called a resectoscope was inserted into the urethra and used to remove excess prostate tissue. The urologist made the gesture of coring an apple. Others were somewhat more invasive, he said, but his experience was that the vast majority of patients with my problems did very well with a TURP.

I thought this over, with Arthur's comments very much in mind. I did not want to say it, but I would do almost anything to ensure that the urologist wasn't given an opportunity to put a resectoscope up my penis and start cutting. What are the aftereffects? I asked. How about retrograde ejaculation, for instance?

He frowned. Where had I picked up that phrase? I gave him a brief account of Arthur's case. He shook his head. Retrograde ejaculation was not a problem to most men, he assured me—the sensation remained pretty much the same. Some even preferred it.

I asked if there were other possible aftereffects. He thought about it. Not really, he said. Some men experience—he paused—"erectile dysfunction." Others, temporary incontinence.

Oh, boy, I thought. Impotence and incontinence! We sat in silence while he tapped his fingers impatiently on his blotter. Were there any nonsurgical treatments? I asked.

He sighed. There were a number of new and relatively untested drugs, he suggested rather unwillingly—his heart was clearly in surgery as the answer to my problem. Hytrin was reputed to "relax" the prostate and take some of the pressure off the urethra. Some patients did well on it. Proscar, though still more or less experimental, actually shrank prostate tissue over the long haul. Of course, both had side effects. Hytrin made some men feel weak, fatigued, even mildly dizzy at times; some patients complained that Proscar reduced or eliminated—he coughed discreetly—"their libido."

I didn't much like the sound of that, but all things considered either drug seemed like a better alternative than surgery, and I left the office with samples of both, having agreed that I would try Hytrin, then move on to Proscar if I experienced difficulties. The urologist looked disappointed.

—⟋⟍—

I WAS NEVER able to test Hytrin's ability to "relax" the prostate—it relaxed *me* so much that I found myself losing consciousness whenever I stood up suddenly. I reported this to my urologist, who remarked that this was certainly a problem with Hytrin. Why hadn't he mentioned it *specifically?*, I wondered, before my knees gave out from under me and I fell on my forehead—and started in on Proscar.

To my astonishment, however, Proscar worked. Not at first, to be sure—it took at least two months before I noticed any improvement—but as time went by all my symptoms declined, then vanished, as if I had visited Lourdes successfully. I no longer needed to look for rest rooms or get up two or three times at night. On the other hand, the warning on the physicians' samples of Proscar (since my experience with Hytrin and Arthur's with the renegade cold medicine I had taken to reading the fine print on all medication) was amply justified. I lost all libido, just as the urologist had said might be the case. It wasn't that I *couldn't* have sex; I simply hadn't any interest at all in doing so—nothing, however provocative, aroused me.

It was a strange feeling—almost monastic. I wasn't sure what I thought about it. For several months I stayed on the Proscar, but in the end I couldn't live with chemical celibacy. Without telling the doctor, I stopped taking it, and—lo and behold!—a miracle occurred. Not only did my libido return, but my prostate stayed shrunk! Against the odds, despite the fact that Proscar is only supposed to be effective for so long as the patient stays on it, I was cured.

I touched wood, but as the months went by there was no denying it—my symptoms were gone. I could pee with perfect ease, without undue pressure, with complete control. Proscar wasn't supposed to work that way, but it had. I decided to find out who manufactured it and buy a few shares of stock.

I made an appointment to have my much-delayed annual physical done, if only to give my long-suffering internist the good news personally.

3

"IT'S LIKE A MIRACLE!" I SAID, SITTING NAKED ON THE EXAMINING table.

My internist nodded as he disposed of his latex glove. "It's certainly very unusual," he said cautiously. "The medication isn't supposed to work that way at all. Of course, there's always a degree of autosuggestion in these things. . . ."

But I wasn't prepared to have my internist rain on my parade. I felt completely fine, for the first time in years, and Proscar had done it. He drew a blood sample. "We'll get the usual readings," he said. "I don't suppose there'll be any problems, but you can't be too careful. . . . Of course, you're at the age when your PSA level is getting important."

I raised an eyebrow. What was that? I asked. The PSA test, he explained, is done to determine the *likelihood* of prostate cancer. He showed a certain skepticism about it—a high number, he said, did not necessarily prove that tumors were present; a low number was no guarantee that they weren't. It wasn't, he emphasized, infallible. For that reason, both the British and the French medical societies were strongly opposed to PSA testing on a large scale, and even in this country it was controversial as a screening test, though it was believed to have a certain value as a precaution.

This seemed to me a little strange. What, after all, is the point of a test which may or may not prove anything? And why hadn't I had it done before? I asked.

He sighed. I *had* had it done before. It was one of the many items on my annual blood test. If he had not mentioned it—and he was pretty sure he had—that was because the results had always been within normal parameters. .

With what *had been* the normal parameters, he corrected himself. The problem was, he went on, that "they" kept dropping the number at which the patient's PSA level was cause for alarm. He did not say who "they" were, but he was clearly irritated by them. Formerly anything below 10 was considered safe enough. Now the threshold was said to be at 4 or 5! Who knew what it might be a year or two from now? His expression showed the exasperation of a practical physician for pie-in-the-sky theorists who came up with ever more demanding tests: "they," I guessed.

Since he had already proclaimed his satisfaction with my prostate after his DRE (the dreaded sound of a latex glove snapping again!), I did not pay much attention to a test in which he himself seemed to have very little confidence, nor did I ask him what my PSA level had been the last time it was taken. He had probed the organ with his finger and found nothing. If that was good enough for him, it was plenty good enough for me.

I left his office with that feeling of satisfaction—and virtue—that comes from having done the sensible thing and had my annual physical on time instead of putting it off, all the more so since my internist had passed me with flying colors—subject to the results of my blood test, about which he hadn't expressed the slightest concern.

As I walked down Madison Avenue on the way to my office I felt a glow of good health warming me, despite a chill wind that had everybody else tightening their mufflers and pulling up their overcoat collars. There was vigor in my every stride. I congratulated myself on my good fortune—and on having always taken good care of myself: skipping rich desserts, avoiding fatty foods, drinking decaffeinated coffee, using margarine instead of butter (this was before "they" discovered that margarine causes cancer and that butter is healthier). I drank alcohol moderately, and had given up smoking a pipe nearly five years before.

My sixtieth birthday was coming up the following year, but people were always telling me—even my doctor, even my *wife*—that I looked years younger.

Glancing at myself in the shop windows, I thought they were right. Except for my prostate I was in great shape, and now even that was no longer troubling me.

I congratulated myself. I was a lucky man.

———

MY GOOD LUCK lasted all of twenty-four hours. The next morning, while I was sipping my decaffeinated, skimmed-milk cappuccino with one packet of Equal—what could be healthier?—the telephone on my desk rang and I picked it up. It was my internist.

If I had been paying more attention, I might have noticed a certain grimness in his voice, but I was still coasting on a health high. "Everything's fine," he said. A pause. "The only thing I don't like is the result of the PSA test."

I reminded myself what the PSA test was, and felt a certain chill. What's the number?, I asked.

"Fifteen," he said.

I recalled that 10 had once been considered the threshold beyond which the presence of cancer was a possibility. Then "they" had decreed that the safe level was below 4 or 5. Even by the *old* standards I was well above the danger level; by the new ones, my PSA was at least three times higher than it should have been.

"Just how bad is this news?" I asked.

He coughed. "It might not mean a damn thing, frankly," he said. "Don't get upset about it. Not yet, anyway. The prostate felt normal enough to me. Sometimes people with enlarged prostates like yours run very high numbers—much higher than this—without any sign of cancer at all. Any kind of prostate infection can make the number spike. It can spike for no reason at all."

"I see." I wasn't sure whether to be relieved or anxious.

"Of course, you should go back and see the urologist again. He'll want to do some tests, just as a precaution."

That caught my attention. "What *kind* of tests?" I asked. "Is there a lot of pain involved?" I kicked myself for sounding like a wimp. I approach a routine colonoscopy as one might a firing squad, and it generally requires so much Valium to get me through one that I need to be carried home afterward, as limp as a rag doll. The memory of the urologist's unsmiling face made me pretty sure that whatever urology had in store for me in the way of "tests" was likely to be even less appealing.

"Pain? No, no, don't worry about it. He'll do an ultrasound of the prostate. That's nothing. If he sees anything suspicious, he'll probably take a biopsy. That's no big deal, either."

"So if the ultrasound is okay, he *won't* do a biopsy, is that right?" I asked, clinging to this frail hope. I didn't know much, but I could guess that taking a tissue sample out of the prostate, given where it was, was likely to be right up there with a colonoscopy on the discomfort scale.

"Mmm," he said.

———

My SWEATY ANXIETY about having a biopsy taken made my urologist raise an eyebrow.

Like my internist, he too felt it was no big deal. Following his nurse's instructions, I had given myself a Fleet enema in the evening, and again in the morning, a process not calculated to raise my spirits.

No sooner was I undressed, and the ritual DRE completed (*snap!* went the latex glove again), than the urologist proceeded with his ultrasound examination of my prostate, which I watched with a certain fearful curiosity. The ultrasound probe looked like the end of an old-fashioned bedpost, and was so large that it resembled the kind of monstrous dildo that is generally featured in books like *Story of O* or the works of the Marquis de Sade. Once it was inserted into my posterior, I was able to see my prostate on what looked like a radar screen, a blob of dark and light patches, which the doctor studied silently, frowning. I felt a certain discomfort, but no pain—indeed, I congratulated myself for my bravery under fire.

"How does it look?" I asked him.

He peered at the screen. "I see no cause for alarm so far," he said. "Of course, the biopsies will tell us a lot more."

I felt a chill that went beyond what is natural to a man lying half naked on a cold examination table covered in paper, with an ultrasound probe up his ass. "I thought you only went ahead with the biopsy if the ultrasound shows a problem."

Out of the corner of one eye I could see his nurse busying herself with what looked like a piece of industrial equipment about two feet long, with a wicked-looking spring-loaded cutting tool at the end of a long, flexible probe. Unreasonably, I felt betrayed.

The urologist turned away from the screen reluctantly. "I don't know where you got that idea," he said. "The biopsy is just an extension of the ultrasound. The two procedures are linked. In layman's terms, we use the ultrasound to guide the needle. It's all quite simple."

Layman—the most insulting word in a doctor's vocabulary. I swallowed my annoyance. "Is the procedure, ah, painful?" I asked, conscious of sounding like a layman again—worse still, a timorous one. I couldn't help it. Somehow, I felt that if I *knew* it was going to be painful, I could prepare myself for what was inevitably going to happen in a few moments—unless, that is, I removed the ultrasound probe, stood up, and walked out, a fantasy that occupied my mind for a second or two.

He chuckled. "Painful?" he said. "Not for me."

He inserted the probe. "You'll hear a click each time I pull the trigger," he said. "There'll be a *pulling* sensation, then a quick pinch—nothing to be excited about at all."

I heard the click, and felt a quick stab, followed by shame at my own cowardice.

"There," he said cheerfully. "I told you it was nothing. It'll be a lot easier if you just relax."

I nodded. Relax? How, I asked myself, was I to relax while lying on my side, vulnerable and half naked, while a doctor probed deep into my prostate, snipping off tiny plugs of tissue as a gardener might cut flowers? I forced my mind elsewhere, and reminded myself that the pain was a lot less severe, in fact, than a root canal or a torn rotator cuff. I counted the clicks, and breathed a sigh relief at the last one. It wasn't so much the pain, I decided, as the position—and the feeling of helplessness.

I wondered why the procedure was done without Valium or any form of anesthetic, and was later (too late, alas) informed that some doctors *do* give their patients something to relax them before the procedure. Knowing this, I strongly recommend your asking for it—*insisting* on it, even—should you ever find yourself in this situation.

When it was over, I cleaned myself up and dressed, thinking, as usual, that I had made a fuss over nothing—an opinion which, I suspect, the doctor shared. Still, as I left his office, bearing a prescription for antibiotics, I had the virtuous feeling that comes from having followed everybody's good advice and done the sensible, grown-up, cautious thing. I felt no anxiety at all—simply relief that it was over and done with.

Less than two days later, I got the good news: the biopsies had proved negative for cancer.

4

WITHIN A WEEK, HOWEVER, I DEVELOPED AN INFECTION FROM THE procedure that dogged me on and off for the next two or three months and which seemed to resist every antibiotic known to man. The summer dragged by and still I felt nothing but soreness and discomfort, far worse in some ways than what I had experienced during the period of my prostate problems. I was uncomfortable driving long distances, even *short* distances; I took to carrying about a foam rubber pillow again; I bought medical sheepskins to sit on, one for home, one for the office, one for the car. Sitting became a problem unless I was cushioned like the Princess and the Pea.

My urologist was reluctant to admit that his biopsy had caused this long bout of infection but could find no other explanation. Eventually, having wasted a summer during which I was pretty much immobilized by constant discomfort and the side effects of innumerable antibiotics, I found the condition waning. As the snows returned I began to feel well again.

Along the way, I had picked up from friends and total strangers a wealth of remedies for prostate trouble. I drank cranberry juice morning, noon, and night, as well as enough Evian water to float the battleship *Missouri,* not to speak of evil-smelling herb teas. Following the advice of Margaret's masseur, I took a daily smorgasbord of capsules: zinc, potassium, selenium, antioxidants, aloe vera. I ate freeze-dried organic bee pollen by the spoonful. As a part-time resident of Santa Fe, New Mexico, I sought out herbal and root concoctions at the local *botanicas* recommended by Margaret's manicurist, and was also provided with a list of Chinese remedies, not easily found even at the Good Earth, Santa Fe's huge health-food supermarket, with names like Tiger Drops and puzzling directions for dosage.

It wasn't that I was becoming a hypochondriac—I felt fine and I wasn't worried—but I was looking for *insurance* against the return of my problems. After all, how much harm could a few foul-tasting drops of saw palmetto extract do, or a sprinkling of bee pollen on my cereal? None at all, I told myself, and it was probably true—though the *real* truth was that I would do anything, take anything, in order not to see the urologist again. I was better, and determined to stay that way.

The only trouble was that despite all the health food, the cranberry juice, and the Chinese homeopathic medicine, I found myself getting more and more tired.

—◦—

I FOUND A thousand ways to deny my fatigue, and even more ways to hide it or excuse it to myself. After all, I kept to a busy work schedule and a rigorous exercise schedule. Why *shouldn't* I be tired from time to time? But it wasn't a comfortable kind of tiredness, the kind that comes at the end of a busy day or an exciting evening, the kind you get when you've had a good run or a hard workout, with a pleasant ache in the joints that responds to a hot bath and a drink, and promises a solid eight hours of sleep. This was more like slamming quite suddenly, at unpredictable moments in the day, into a brick wall. I found myself stretching out on my couch in the office after lunch for a brief nap—not at all my usual pattern. I, who usually walked at a rapid pace, occasionally felt that simply putting one foot in front of another was all I could manage—even *more* than I could manage, often.

Once I found myself literally *stuck* in the middle of Forty-ninth Street, halfway down the block, unable to summon up the energy to move forward toward my lunch date, and seriously doubtful that I could make it back to my office, less than a hundred yards behind me. Strange changes were taking place in my life. Formerly I was always awake far later than Margaret, and up at the crack of dawn to read or write. Now I was in bed and asleep long before her, and often finding reasons for sleeping later.

I persuaded myself that it was nothing. I needed a change, I decided. I needed more exercise (or perhaps less). I increased my intake of vitamin C until my urine was a bright buttercup yellow, and I added E, B, and A until the kitchen countertop resembled a pharmacy. None of it did the least bit of good—when fatigue hit me, it hit like a ton of bricks.

The winter passed, spring came, my prostate remained quiescent, but now it was fatigue, more and more, that got in the way of my doing what I wanted to do. By the summer, I could no longer deny that *something* was wrong.

I complained to my internist, but he could find nothing wrong. I should take a vacation, he told me—I should learn to relax. But I couldn't relax, and I was too tired to even think about taking a vacation, let alone actually travel somewhere. At regular intervals I went back to my internist and we tried to identify the source of my fatigue, but nothing came of it. I was 100 percent fit and totally wiped out.

October brought a moment of excitement that overcame my increasing weariness. We celebrated my sixtieth birthday with a glamorous bash at Tavern on the Green. It was Margaret's birthday present to me, and she turned it into a memorable extravaganza, with Penthouse Pet Amy Lynn jumping out of a real cake, icing and all, strolling Gypsy violinists, a gourmet banquet, and, as a special surprise, a short film documenting my life. Nearly two hundred guests—some of them friends I hadn't seen for nearly twenty years—drank, danced, and gave speeches. Margaret had never looked more beautiful, and in the heady glow of affection and celebration I regained my energy.

The high of my birthday receded, and gradually the periods of fatigue returned. The winter crept by, spring and summer came, and while I never felt really *bad*, I didn't feel quite *right*, either. I couldn't put my finger on the problem, couldn't even describe it for my doctor, whose only suggestion was that I should take some time off—go to a Club Med, he told me, spend a week on one of the islands, sit on the beach, *relax*.

He was beginning to sound to me more like a travel agent than a doctor. What I wanted was a prescription, or at the very least a diagnosis, not travel advice. And even if I had *wanted* to follow his advice, I didn't have the energy to plan, pack, travel. People who knew me well thought I looked tired and drawn, noticed that I was prone to the kind of irritation and bursts of temper that accompany fatigue, sometimes even complained about it. Things that would normally have interested me—invitations to appear on television, or to write a short piece for a magazine or newspaper, or to go to a party—seemed like too much trouble to accept.

I was uneasily conscious, too, that I had let more than a year go by since my last PSA test. I kept putting it off, from week to week, not out of fear, but simply because I didn't want to do anything that might result in my having to visit the urologist again.

So far as my prostate was concerned, I was determined to let sleeping dogs lie.

———

AUTUMN CAME. WE made plans to go to Santa Fe for Thanksgiving and Christmas, I cleared the decks to start work on a *New Yorker* piece, I made notes for a new book. Finally, I bit the bullet and made an appointment with my internist for a full physical, just about eighteen months since the last one, when my PSA had been 15.

I wasn't worried. My biopsy had shown me to be cancer-free, despite the elevated PSA, which both the urologist and my internist had attributed to prostate enlargement. Since then, thanks to Proscar or sheer dumb luck, my prostate was no longer giving me trouble.

When he phoned the next day, though, I knew something was wrong right away. "It's 22 plus," he said, the concern in his voice apparent. The notion that PSA was an unreliable test and that the numbers didn't necessarily mean anything seemed to have flown out the window, judging by the sound of his voice. He was no longer recommending a trip to the Caribbean.

"That's a big jump, isn't it?" I asked. I was doing the numbers rapidly in my head. It was a 50 percent leap in a year and a half, as a matter of fact, more than six times the current "safe" number.

"It is."

"Does that mean I need another biopsy?"

"I'm afraid so."

"Last time around, I hated it. And I got sick."

"That can happen. But you need to be tested."

"Can I put it off until we're back from Santa Fe? There's no point in going all the way out there if I'm feeling really rotten, the way I did after the last biopsy."

"When are you planning to go?"

"Just before Thanksgiving."

There was a long pause. "I wouldn't want you to wait that long," he said.

"Oh." I didn't like the sound of that.

"The sooner the better," he said firmly. "Within reason."

I called my urologist, with infinite reluctance, to make an appointment, only to discover that he was on vacation—I had a vision of him in the Caribbean, which, apparently, served doctors as the equivalent of Lourdes. I was offered the name of a urologist who substituted for him, then it occurred to me to ask a doctor friend what *she* thought I should do.

What she thought, and in no uncertain terms, was that I should go to Memorial Sloan-Kettering's Prostate Cancer Detection Center as soon as possible. She called back within an hour to tell me that I had an appointment with Dr. Peter Russo for the next Tuesday.

Since she had warned me that it might take from six to eight weeks to get an appointment, I was suitably impressed with her clout—though, had my head been screwed on the right way, I might also have drawn the conclusion that a rise in my PSA from 15 to 22 was the oncological equivalent of a fire alarm going off.

Happily, this thought did not occur to me.

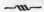

It was thus that I found myself a few days later, on a Tuesday morning, in the calm, elegant, and even luxurious waiting room of Memorial Sloan-Kettering's Prostate Cancer Detection Center, accompanied this time by Margaret, who, knowing my fear of the biopsy, had come along to hold my hand so long as she was allowed to.

Thankfully, the Prostate Cancer Detection Center is not actually *in* Memorial Sloan-Kettering Hospital, but is several blocks away. Hospitals are frightening, I find, and a hospital devoted entirely to cancer is particularly so. Somebody had decided to make sure that this place *wasn't* frightening, and done a pretty good job of it.

The Prostate Cancer Detection Center fills a small, modern building with lots of big windows. From the outside, it looks like the Upper East Side office of a trendy architect or designer; inside, the soothing gray and off-white color scheme, modern furniture, and thriving plants seem designed to put the visitor at his ease. Even the reading material was up-to-date, despite medical tradition that magazines in any hospital waiting area must be two-year-old copies of *Prevention* and *Reader's Digest*.

Dr. Russo, I discovered when Margaret and I were taken to an examining room, was young, good-looking, and intense; his associate (I thought of him as Russo's "sidekick"), Dr. Fleishner, was tall, bespectacled, smiling, relaxed. Like the traditional "good cop–bad cop" combination, they seemed total opposites, though there was no doubt that Russo was the one in charge. Both looked serious when I mentioned my PSA. Here at Memorial Sloan-Kettering, they made it clear, there were no doubts at all about whether the PSA reading really meant something.

Only later was I to discover that Russo is a distinguished urological surgeon, a superstar of the scalpel in his own right. I'm glad I didn't know this at the time. There's something inherently discomforting about the fact that in urology most biopsies for prostate cancer are performed by surgeons. Perhaps it doesn't matter that surgeons, obviously, make their living by performing surgery—though, as I was later to discover, a lot of patients feel hustled into the operating room unnecessarily, in the doctor's interests rather than their own—but it certainly *does* matter that a surgeon's instinctive bias is, naturally, toward cutting.

Surgeons, not surprisingly, believe that surgery is the best way to solve a problem, which can only color their view of alternative treatments, whether conventional, like hormone therapy or radiology, or experimental, like cryoablation (in which the affected parts of the prostate are frozen).

Admittedly, surgery may often be the best answer to prostate cancer, provided the patient is neither too old nor the cancer too far advanced; and also admittedly, the best urologists are usually willing to *discuss* alternative treatments, albeit with a degree of scorn—still, it's a little as if the umpire were also playing in the game.

Happily, in my innocence I was spared any of these concerns. Far from being worried about surgery, I was only concerned about the brief pain (referred to by urologists as "discomfort") of the biopsy procedure, which I took to be another formality. When I wistfully mentioned that I was afraid of the biopsy, having had a difficult experience with it eighteen months before, Dr. Russo turned from his examination of the ultrasound pictures of my prostate, grabbed my shoulder, and told me, in a strong, passionate voice, that if I were his own brother he would urge me to have it done.

I went next door with Dr. Fleishner, who did the procedure quickly, efficiently, and with a lot less pain than my urologist had managed. He also took a lot more biopsies, ten rather than six. I asked him about this.

"It's just to be on the safe side," he said cheerfully. He made it clear that at Memorial Sloan-Kettering they prided themselves on being thorough, probing far deeper into the prostate than most urologists would do when taking a biopsy. "If there are tumors present," he told me, "we find them. If we give you a clean bill of health, it's *clean*."

Just my luck, I thought. I've come to the one place in New York where they take *more* samples than my own urologist does. But Dr. Fleishner was so jolly that in the end I didn't mind it.

I would be given the results of the biopsies on Thursday, Dr. Fleishner told me, with a ritual snap of his latex gloves. Kathy would call me.

I dressed and rejoined Margaret in the waiting room, thankful that the worst was over, and grateful that it hadn't been as bad as I'd expected.

That was it, for another year or so, I told myself, with a sigh of relief.

I didn't give Thursday a thought.

5

BUT OF COURSE THURSDAY TURNED OUT TO BE SOMETHING OF A landmark day in my life: The Day I Discovered I Had Cancer.

Looking back on it, I could see a lot of signs that I should have paid more attention to—that *somebody* should have paid more attention to, anyway: the fatigue, the urinary problems, the simple, deep-down feeling that *something* was wrong.

I had always made fun of those well-meaning friends, recent converts to health food, or yoga, or some other fad, who were always warning, "You should listen to your body."

My concern had always been more along the lines of getting my body to listen to *me*, a natural preoccupation for a man in his sixties, when all sorts of functions that used to take place at will begin to present difficulties. Yet I could now see, quite clearly, that my body *had* indeed been trying to catch my attention, to warn me that something was dreadfully, dangerously wrong, and I had stoutly refused to listen.

The unpleasant truth about most cancers is that they have usually been present in one's body for a long time before they're discovered, and that the body, terrified at the first approach of a killer, has been dialing 911 frantically and getting no reply. Most of us are too frightened of the possibility of having cancer to pay any heed. Thus, many men ignore changes in their urinary habits, discomfort, and a host of other warnings, and don't turn up at the urologist's office until they have noticed blood in their urine or crippling aches and pains in the back, at which point, all too often, cancer has metastasized to the bone, and successful treatment is highly unlikely.

It gradually began to dawn on me that had I gone to the Memorial Sloan-Kettering Prostate Cancer Detection Center eighteen months before for my biopsy, they might well have found cancer then. What Russo and Fleishner were telling me, in the indirect way in which physicians comment on their colleagues, was that when a sixty-year-old man appeared before them with a PSA that had risen from 15 to 22 in eighteen months, their presumption was that he had prostate cancer, and the challenge would be to *find* it—hence the numerous "deep" biopsies. Far from being a doubtful test, for *these* doctors, who specialized in prostate cancer, the PSA number was the Holy Grail. They had not been "looking" for cancer—they knew it was there, and were prepared to keep on digging until they found it.

As I was to discover, the dispute about how much attention should be paid to PSA—a dispute which actually reached the front page of *The New York Times*—is not an abstract or theoretical one; on the contrary, it is a question of life or death for many men. Given the fact that most prostate cancers are asymptomatic (that is, that they produce no symptoms) and that PSA is a fairly reliable indicator of whether cancer is present in the prostate or not—and even, to a degree, how far advanced it may be—one would suppose that the medical establishment and the government would be beating the drums to make every man over forty aware of the need to be tested, as has been the case for mammograms. Women can hardly open a newspaper, or a magazine, or watch television without being urged to have a regular mammogram, and one might suppose that it might make good sense to have male stars and authority figures urging men to get their PSA taken on a regular basis.

But no, on the contrary; PSA has been explicitly *rejected* as a "screening" test. Doctors argue that "most" men over fifty or sixty have cancer cells present in their prostate but will probably die of something else. The tumors are often very small, the disease is usually slow-growing, no treatment is called for—so why alarm the patient about something which doesn't threaten his life expectancy? On the average, it takes at least ten to twelve years for prostate cancer to metastasize sufficiently to kill the patient, and sometimes more, so for many men older than sixty-five, life expectancy with prostate cancer is about the same as it would be *without* prostate cancer.

Besides, so this argument goes, if every man over a certain age were tested regularly for PSA, as women are for breast cancer, tens of thousands, perhaps *hundreds* of thousands, of men would be demanding treatment for a condition which may require, in the vast majority of cases, only "watchful waiting," while hospitals would be swamped by men undergoing treatment for tiny, slow-growing tumors that don't require any treatment at all, least of all expensive major surgery. The cost would be astronomical.

This is the factor which has made the French and the British medical establishments skeptical of widespread PSA testing, and which concerns health-care plans and insurance companies in the United States. It is one of the many reasons why prostate cancer doesn't get anything like the amount of attention, research money, or publicity that breast cancer does—the other being, perhaps, that while women have learned to band together when it comes to their health concerns, men don't see themselves as a *group,* even when it comes to such male concerns as heart disease and prostate cancer.

The fact is, of course, that while many men *do* have microscopic tumors that will never threaten their lives, and while prostate cancer *is* usually slow-growing, particularly in older men, it can also spread with remarkable speed, and once it *has* spread beyond the prostate capsule there is no stopping it except by drastic measures that will almost certainly have a major impact on the patient's "quality of life."

Playing down the dangers of prostate cancer seems an odd and paradoxical approach to the disease—it is not hard to guess what an outcry there would be if doctors pooh-poohed the dangers of breast cancer, for instance, or sought reasons why it was too expensive to screen large numbers of women for it.

Oncologists, on the whole, take a less ambiguous view of prostate cancer. For them, cancer is cancer—by definition, dangerous and life-threatening. With some exceptions—men over seventy, for example—they take the view that if you have a malignancy, it makes sense to remove it if you can. In the case of prostate cancer, unlike many other cancers, the tumors *can* be removed—provided they are diagnosed early enough—by means of a radical prostatectomy, before they can grow or spread.

A few minutes with Drs. Russo and Fleishner at Memorial Sloan-Kettering, before I even *knew* I had cancer, was enough to tell me that *these* guys took cancer seriously. It was not a question of scaring me—their concern spoke for itself. Cancer is a killer, period—that might as well have been the motto of the Prostate Cancer Detection Center. There was no talk here about how slow-growing prostate cancer was, or how practically every American man over the age of forty had microscopic cancer cells in his prostate. The presence of cancer sounded the alarm, clear and loud.

—◊—

I HEARD IT even in the gentle Kathy's voice, as she gave me the bad news that Thursday afternoon in 1994. If you have any plans, her voice made it clear, forget about them. In case I had any doubts about it (and I didn't), my first priority was cancer and the tests needed to determine whether it was already killing me—the MRI and the bone scan, in particular; for prostate cancer, once it has grown beyond the capsule of the prostate itself, tends to metastasize in the lymph system and the bones, at which point it is no longer curable. Henceforth, it would be the doctors' schedules that would determine what I was going to be doing and when, not mine.

By the middle of the afternoon I had emptied my calendar for the next week or so of appointments that had seemed to me, until only a few minutes before getting the news, of vital importance. An appointment with a bestselling author and his agent would have to be postponed in favor of one with a radiologist; a meeting about my autumn 1995 list of books (would I still be alive in the autumn of 1995?, I found myself wondering dolefully) gave place to a CAT scan. The names and addresses of doctors began to crowd my calendar, though not before I made the discovery that they were far busier than I was, and much harder to reach.

I was apprehensive, not so much about the *results* of the tests, curiously enough, but about the tests themselves, which loomed before me like some dreadful obstacle course. I tried not to think about them for the next week, with only partial success. I read the books I had bought, and learned enough from them to be aware that if my cancer had spread to the bone, the prognosis was poor. None of it felt quite real as yet—my mind simply hadn't accepted the enormous change in my life, from healthy man to cancer patient, perhaps because, as is so typical of prostate cancer, I was totally asymptomatic. I felt fine, I ran or swam every day, I ate and drank normally, even my prostate was quiescent, giving me no trouble at all, now that it was actually pointing a dagger at my heart. Perhaps a better clue to the condition of my subconscious was that I took the trouble to make sure that Margaret had the number of my safe-deposit box.

Almost twenty years before, I had been a daily visitor to Memorial Sloan-Kettering, to see either Cornelius Ryan or Leo Szilard. The memory of it still haunted me. I could remember, only too clearly, the faces of those men I knew so well, bloated from hormones until they were almost unrecognizable, sweating with pain, clinging to life, I thought then, with the arrogance of the young and healthy, long past the point at which it might have been better to let go. Now I wondered how I myself might feel in that same position. Would *I* want to hang on to the bitter end, or let go?

I felt a certain doleful irony in my situation—life was taking me exactly where I had always feared to go, with exactly the disease I had always been afraid to have.

6

IN THE EVENT, I DIDN'T FIND MY EXPERIENCE AT MEMORIAL SLOAN-Kettering frightening at all. From the very first moment, when a nurse asked me what I was there for, and I replied "I have cancer," I realized that this was where I belonged, in a cancer hospital. There was no shock or surprise in her eyes. Why should there be? *Every* patient there had cancer. In a perverse way, I felt at home. Margaret held my hand as we passed through the portal; then I proceeded to fill out the innumerable forms that precede any medical procedure. Formerly I had always been able to ignore the boxes in which you have to check off existing diseases. Now, with a certain pride, I boldly checked off "Cancer."*

Very shortly I was to become used to hearing the word *cancer* pronounced with a smile. The entire staff of Memorial Sloan-Kettering was relentlessly cheerful and smiling, in part, no doubt, as a self-protective measure—a smile is probably the best way of dealing with eight to twelve hours a day of working with people who are suffering from various degrees of pain, fear, and anxiety. *Everybody* I came into contact with was polite, concerned, and cheerful, which probably went a long way to putting me at my ease in surroundings that were more or less guaranteed to have the opposite effect.

It occurred to me that although Americans are alleged to be deeply dissatisfied with their health-care system, almost everybody in that system, however overburdened and underpaid he or she may be, is

---

* For those who still smoke, the question "Have you ever smoked?" when asked in a cancer hospital, as it constantly is, takes on a new sharpness. If anybody reading this book is still smoking, STOP!

remarkably nice. I have been in Mercedes-Benz showrooms where I was treated with less courtesy and fewer smiles.

Of course, it's no fun being tested, not so much because it's painful—hardly any pain is involved, unless it's that almost everybody in the process, however cheerful, has to take a blood sample, which, as I was soon to discover, is something a cancer patient had better get used to mighty fast—as because the machinery is vast, forbidding, threatening, and heavily stickered with radioactive warning labels.

Even that's not really so bad—you can actually get caught up in the mildly futuristic technology of bone scans and MRIs and CAT scans, and if nothing else you're the center of everybody's attention for a brief moment. What is harder to ignore is the presence of the *other* cancer patients (the "real" ones, I felt then, in my innocence, as opposed to myself), spectral forms waiting patiently—or perhaps *not* patiently, who knows?—on gurneys and in wheelchairs, stacked up in a kind of ghastly holding pattern in the halls. With their drab, wrinkled hospital gowns, their tubes and drips, their pale faces, they made it clear to me just what the consequences would be of failing these particular tests. I would be joining them—perhaps even joining those who had an aiming pattern for their radiation drawn in purple ink on their skulls, looking for all the world like skinheads with exotic tattoos. It was not a comforting thought, which made me all the more grateful for the smiles.

LOOKING BACK ON it, I think that day at Memorial Sloan-Kettering was the longest one of my life—certainly the most crucial one. The morning wasn't so bad—endless blood samples, a visit to the nuclear medicine department for an injection of radioactive isotope, an MRI (like being sent to the bottom of the sea in a tightly confining miniature submarine while somebody beats on the outside of the hull with a rubber hammer), a CAT scan, bone X rays. Several fairly nauseating drips and injections were involved, but nothing I couldn't han-

dle. Rated on a scale of discomfort, it was well below an average session with a dentist. Rated on a scale of *fear,* it was quite another story,
of course, if only because behind all the cheerful smiles I could detect
the signs that this was serious business, and possibly about to become
more than that.

A small group of doctors gathered to study what appeared to be
three-dimensional full-color X rays of my skeleton, heads together
and talking in low voices, like the members of a papal conclave, then
went off, bearing the photographs with them, to consult with higher
authority. They did not share their opinions, whatever they were,
with me, but they didn't seem happy.

The technician had already shown me, with some pride, the pictures of my skeleton—could that grotesque, grinning image be
me?—in which I was hard put to develop even a macabre interest. It
wasn't that I was unimpressed by the technology involved, or the
level of her skill; it was simply that I really didn't *want* to see myself
as a skeleton. I could not help noticing, however, a few bright yellow
flare spots on my bones, faint on the left ribs, strong on the left clavicle. I had asked her what they were. "Nothing to worry about," she
replied quickly, but I noticed that she circled them with a bright red
Chinagraph pencil, and that they were the subject of the conclave's
discussions.

I kept my concerns to myself while Margaret had a late lunch at a
nearby diner (I was forbidden to eat anything)—there didn't seem
any point in sharing them at this stage. If the morning had seemed
slow, the afternoon was positively leaden. We sat for what seemed
like hours on one floor, only to be directed later to another, where we
sat again. More blood was taken, by people who seemed unaware of
the previous tests. A former member of the British armed services, I
recognized the drill. It was not just "hurry up and wait"; it was also,
and more important, the rising of a suspicion that something was
wrong, and that nobody was about to tell us what the problem was.

We had been told we would be finished by two P.M. Soon it was
four, then five, the corridors emptied out, we sat alone, except for a

few other forlorn souls who seemed to have lost their way or, perhaps, simply had no place else to go. We occupied a couple of chairs in a vast lobby, where the only other occupants seemed to be homeless people hoping to spend the night. The receptionist (who knew only too well by now who we were) finished her shift and left, to be replaced by another receptionist who didn't know who we were at all. I wondered if Margaret and I were waiting in the right place. When I was assured we were, I wondered if the news was so dire that nobody wanted to break it to me.

I made my way back and forth to the long-suffering receptionist, who was unable to reach anyone who knew about me. By six o'clock I was trying to call people on the *outside* with my cellular phone, asking them to call in and find out what was going on, since on the inside we were in limbo. I went down to the cafeteria, only to find that it, too, had closed—the whole hospital seemed to be emptying out, giving its long corridors and huge, dim waiting areas a grim, deserted look. (Memorial is not one of those hospitals in which money is frittered away on decoration—there, the money goes into medicine and research.)

Finally, a message for us reached the receptionist, from a doctor unknown to us both. We were directed back to the X-ray department (another rush, followed by another interminable wait). A cheerful young man emerged at long last to explain that it was necessary to take the bone X rays all over again. I undressed and put my clothes in a locker (for the umpteenth time that day), and followed him back, as he chatted away to put me at my ease. "Didn't they come out right last time?" I asked.

He laughed as he prepared to insert yet another needle into my arm. He was young and Hispanic, and looked to my eyes more like a street-smart athlete than a skilled medical technician, but he was so deft with the needle that I hardly even felt it go in. The eyes above the bright smile were dark and professionally calm—this guy, I decided, knew what he was doing. He probably knew why he was doing it, too, but he wasn't about to tell me. "They came out, sure," he said. "They want more detail, that's all. Don't you worry. They want the best man on this. I'm the best man."

He didn't say who "they" were—doctors, I presumed. He didn't say why "they" wanted more detail. He didn't have to. My heart sank, despite his good-natured spiel, half rap, half talk-show host. If "they" wanted more detail it was presumably because "they" had seen something they didn't like. Somehow, during the long course of the day, I had held firmly to the notion that I was going to come out of this all right. I had cancer, sure, I had come to accept that, but there was no way I could accept the idea that it might have *spread*. If I hadn't known what "spread" involved before, I sure did now, after a whole day deep in the bowels of Memorial Sloan-Kettering, down in the nuclear-medicine department. "Spread" was what put you outside in the hallway in one of those wheelchairs with a chrome-plated post attached to it for your IV drips, waiting for someone to push you toward your next treatment, or back to your room to recover from the treatment you had just had. "Spread" meant—for by now I had all but memorized Dr. Rous's book—the relentless progression from hormone therapy to radiation, from radiation to chemotherapy, from chemotherapy to strontium injections, the last resort, "palliative" therapy for bone pain at two or three thousand dollars a shot. Mentally, I braced myself for what was to come, and found a certain peace in contemplating the worst.

By seven P.M. Margaret and I were back in a cavernous lobby, sprawled out on leatherette chairs, totally exhausted from tension and waiting. From time to time, I made my way to the receptionist's desk to remind her of my name—she was another new one—but all she could tell me was that our instructions were to wait. So we waited. A couple of families with small children occupied obscure corners of the lobby. From time to time, patients were wheeled slowly past us. It was not a cheerful place to be.

The young oncologist in charge of my case finally appeared, smiling broadly—a good sign, I thought. Untouchably clean in his crisp white coat, like most doctors he appeared to walk at the pace most people run, projecting an image of superhuman busyness. Where, I wondered—and was to wonder a lot in the next few months—did doctors get all their energy from? Was it their training—the famous brutal nonstop demands of internship and residency? Or was it simply that the doctor—so long as he or she is in an office or, better yet, a hospital—is the one person who is always at the center of things? In any event, at the end of a day that had left me—and Margaret—limp, tired, and bedraggled, this doctor, whose day surely had begun hours before ours and involved God only knew what life-and-death decisions, seemed as fresh as a daisy, ready for hours more. He was, in fact, as he made it clear, on his way to look into another case—*he* was not thinking about going home for a drink and dinner—and in a hurry to get there.

He perched on the arm of Margaret's chair and apologized for keeping us so late. There had been some disagreement about my bone scan, he said. He had taken it to the head of the radiology department himself for another opinion. There was some concern about a few light spots on the films. Had I ever broken my ribs or my clavicle? His expression was hard to decipher, for it was the bland smile of a man steering a fine line between saying something that might frighten the patient and offering false hope.

I remembered the bright spots on my X rays that the technician had circled in red, and understood instantly why the day had dragged on for so long. "I broke my collarbone about twenty years ago," I said. I had, in fact, been thrown from Margaret's old thoroughbred, Tabasco, early one morning in Central Park. For weeks afterward, we had to make love with me lying on my back. As for Tabasco, he went on to a long and happy life, but I never rode him again. He was a big chestnut gelding off the track, handsome and very fast, and he didn't like being ridden by men, though he was a real pussycat in the hands of a pretty woman. I could see his point, and never held my broken shoulder against him.

He nodded. "What about the ribs?"

"I got thrown from a horse again, three or four years ago. I didn't think I'd broken any ribs, but they were mighty sore." Actually, I thought at the time that I'd broken my neck when I landed and was going to have to spend the rest of my life in a wheelchair, so I hadn't taken much notice of the ribs.

"Maybe you should stay off horses."

"My other hobby is motorcycles. Horses are safer."

He smiled. "Well, if that's the case, you're clean. Fractures show up on the pictures the same way as bone cancer does, you see, so there was some concern . . ."

He gave a gentle sigh, and we sat quietly for a moment, the three of us. No doubt, he was relieved that he didn't have to tell me that there were signs that cancer had metastasized to my bones; I was relieved that I had a perfectly sound explanation for the areas of my bone structure that were lit up like Christmas tree ornaments on the X rays.*

The lobby was darkened now. Cleaning people were beginning to sweep up a busy day's worth of trash. "You're very lucky," the doctor said soberly. Then he was on his feet again, as tensed up and eager to get moving to his next case as a runner on his blocks.

We shook hands briskly. "Of course, the sooner you can get your surgery scheduled, the better," he said. "When are you seeing Dr. Russo?"

"Tuesday afternoon."

"Great! He's a good man. You can't go wrong."

"Should I get a second opinion?"

His face was thoughtful. Dr. Russo was his colleague. Institutional loyalty is strong among doctors, stronger, I think, than in any other profession except the Marines. For this oncologist, Memorial Sloan-Kettering came first, last, and always. "You might want to do that,"

---

* I was only later—much later—to discover just how relieved I should have been. In fact, the day had been prolonged by the fear that the cancer had indeed spread, to the point of being incurable, and the oncologist had finally taken my X rays to the head of the radiology department himself, who had given me a clean bill of health provided the bright spots could be explained. It was probably just as well that I did not know how close I was to the grimmest kind of bad news that afternoon. I am still grateful for the care and attention that I received that day, and for the special effort that was made to get me results in one day, rather than having to wait for them.

he said cautiously. "Russo's a first-class surgeon. There are other good surgeons out there, of course. . . . Lots of people aren't happy until they've seen Pat Walsh, down at Johns Hopkins, for example. . . ." He gave a smile that seemed to suggest I wasn't necessarily that kind of person. "It's really up to you."

With that, he told us to go out and celebrate, and rushed back to work.

I wondered who Pat Walsh was.

7

"I'D LIE DOWN IN FRONT OF THE TAXI THAT'S TAKING YOU TO THE hospital to stop you from going to anyone except Pat Walsh!" Ken Aretsky said fervently.

Aretsky, a successful restaurateur and a comparative stranger, had called me out of the blue, an act of genuine kindness, to offer me his advice. I was touched.

He was not alone, however. From the moment the word was out that I had prostate cancer, I came to realize how true the words "misery loves company" are. Cocooned in my illusion of good health, it had escaped my attention that Senator Robert Dole, General Norman Schwarzkopf, Sidney Poitier, and Roger Moore (not to mention my barber and two of my neighbors in the country) had all had prostate cancer. I could hardly believe how many people I knew who either *had* prostate cancer or knew someone who did. My telephone rang day and night with friends, acquaintances, and total strangers, all of them eager to give me advice, most of it sharply conflicting: I must absolutely have surgery, the sooner, the better; I must not even *think* of having surgery—radiation was the only way to go; I should avoid surgery and radiation at all costs, and go for hormone therapy instead; I should avoid *all* the conventional treatments and try cryoablation, a revolutionary new procedure in which the tumors in the prostate are frozen with liquid nitrogen; I should do nothing at all, and merely follow the "watchful waiting" protocol that was the rule in the United Kingdom and France, having my PSA checked every couple of months. . . .

Through all this mass of well-meant and conflicting information (and misinformation, as I was soon to discover) there was one piece of advice that came up again and again, a kind of leitmotif that kept repeating itself: Whatever I was going to do, I should seek a consultation first with Pat Walsh.

Dr. Patrick C. Walsh of Johns Hopkins was, it appeared, the superstar of prostate-cancer surgery, the inventor of the "nerve-sparing" technique for radical prostatectomy (about which much, *much* more later), the guru and doyen of urology. His name was uttered with awe by everyone, even other doctors, although they always mentioned him with a certain amount of envy. Everyone, even those in the anti-surgery camp, invoked his name.

I put Dr. Walsh's name firmly in the back of my mind—*far* in the back—conscious that I had not yet had my consultation with Dr. Russo. To those who wanted me to fly down to Baltimore on the next airplane in the hope that Dr. Walsh might have a last-minute cancellation or who offered to call him on my behalf, I replied—sensibly, I thought—that I could hardly seek a second opinion when I had not yet had the first one.

The truth was that I still harbored the illusion that surgery might not be called for, and that Russo, when I saw him, might suggest some less invasive alternative.

—◦—

EVERYBODY WANTED TO help. I was constantly urged to talk to this or that person who had had a radical prostatectomy and was either "as good as new" or "better than ever." An extraordinary number of women in the book business seemed to have fathers who had gone through the same thing I was enduring, and who had recovered from it completely.

The fact was, I didn't really *want* to hear the intimate details of some stranger's operation—an operation that I was still hoping to avoid—but I also didn't want to be thought rude and unfeeling, particularly of my fellow cancer sufferers.

Unfortunately, most of what I heard when I did return these calls was less than confidence-inspiring. Their nearest and dearest might believe that they were doing fine, but many of the men I talked to had plenty of complaints, most of them having to do with incontinence and impotence, and discussed them with me even though I was a total stranger.

One of my authors, who had been asked to cheer me up, ended by whispering to me that he was still totally impotent four months after surgery and was seeing a therapist about it. I knew, of course, as Dr. Rous's book made very clear, that the return of erections after even the most "successful" of nerve-sparing radical prostatectomies was unlikely to take place until at least six months or a year after surgery, though there were rare exceptions, of course, like William Martin and his nine-day resurgence.

Feeling a little strange as we reversed roles—this time with me as the comforter—I quoted Dr. Rous's opinion to my author. "You're kidding," he said, obviously relieved that there was still hope for him. To my surprise, he hadn't read Rous's book—or any other book, for that matter—nor had his surgeon spoken to him at all on the subject of sex. He had been sent home after major surgery, without any information, to sweat out by himself one of the more difficult problems that can face a sexually active man.

Even *good* news, I discovered, was often not quite as good as it sounded at first. Not everyone dealt well with "partial" erections or "dry" orgasms (for the surgery removed the seminal vesicles along with the prostate). I soon realized that those who called offering advice were all too often in need of a sympathetic listener themselves, caught up in a silent, lonely misery I hadn't ever known about, and about which, all too often, their wives were the very people they *couldn't* talk to, out of shame or the simple inability to deal with what they perceived as sexual failure.

Still, they confirmed that Dr. Rous was apparently on target in his book. *Good* news after a radical prostatecomy was a partial erection and resumption of intercourse after a year or so; *bad* news, in this area, didn't take much imagination to guess at. I tried not to think too much about it, but I was beginning to understand, for the first time and all too well, why a large number of men, faced with prostate cancer, do nothing.

I thought about the importance sexual intercourse had always had in my life, and tried to imagine what life would be like without it. It seemed like a bleak prospect. Nor was it just a risk of surgery. Radiotherapy, hormone therapy, even cryoablation, all carried the same risk—or, if Dr. Rous was to be believed, a higher risk—of impotence. There was apparently *no* way to get rid of prostate cancer that did not involve some risk of impotence, temporary or permanent, not to speak of some degree of incontinence.

And yet, I reflected, people survived, got on with their lives, beat the odds, learned other forms of eroticism, or simply learned to live happily with their loss. The thing to remember, always, was that this was *cancer,* I told myself, though without much conviction. As one of my doctor friends told me, with cold realism, "It's war: if you don't kill it, it will kill you."

—⁓—

THE METAPHOR OF cancer as warfare came up frequently—it is hardly surprising that oncologists sometimes refer to themselves as being "in the trenches" (as opposed to doctors in more effete specialties), or that patients are said to be fighting a winning or a losing "battle" against cancer, for there is, surrounding cancer treatment, a faint taste of World War I, of heroic attacks against overwhelming odds, of terrible losses and unspeakable suffering, of hand-to-hand fighting against a powerful enemy. For make no mistake about it, cancer is personalized, with good reason, as the *enemy:* cunning, swift-moving, deadly, giving no quarter, taking no prisoners. If you've got it, get rid of it, is the best advice; but getting rid of it, even when possible, is all too frequently a brutal business: a battle.

It is no accident that surgeons refer to the site of the operation as "the field," as in "battlefield" or "field of fire." A radical prostatectomy is warlike surgery. You get rid of the cancer by removing the organ it has "invaded." With any luck, *if* it hasn't yet spread to the surface of the prostate or beyond, you have beaten the enemy. QED.

Simple truth: to defeat cancer you have to destroy a part of yourself. Surgery removes tissue. Radiation destroys tissue. Chemotherapy does all sorts of damage to organs and tissue. Whatever way you attack the cancer, you can't kill it without sacrificing some part of yourself, just as no commander can expect to attack the enemy without taking losses. At some point in the process, the surgeon and/or the radiologist reaches a limit where the patient can no longer sacrifice organs, flesh, *self.* Then other tactics or various palliative treatments may be called upon in an effort to produce "a truce" with the enemy— "stalemate," as opposed to unconditional victory or abject defeat. But until that point is reached, the only question is how much of himself the prostate-cancer patient is prepared (or able) to sacrifice to get rid of the cancer, he hopes once and for all. Victory doesn't come cheaply, or easily, and anybody who tells you different is lying.

—⁂—

A GOOD FRIEND put me in touch with a man who had recently recovered from prostate-cancer surgery at the hands of (who else?) Pat Walsh. This man was a busy CEO who rearranged his schedule in order to take me to lunch the next day, determined to make sure I understood that prostate cancer is *dangerous,* that I had to take it seriously.

If this seems like unnecessary advice, it's not. Most men diagnosed as having prostate cancer feel absolutely fine, as I did, and are all too frequently in the best of health otherwise. Once you know the cancer hasn't spread, it is tempting to put off surgery, to search for alternative treatments, to avoid exposing oneself to the risks of incontinence and impotence, as well as the pain and problems that inevitably accompany major surgery.

Seymour, the CEO, had no doubts. He was a true believer, absolutely determined that I *have* the surgery and that I go to Pat Walsh at Johns Hopkins for it. Like Ken Aretsky, he was willing, even eager, to lie down in front of whatever vehicle might take me to any other hospital than Johns Hopkins, or deliver me into anybody else's hands than Walsh's.

He was not alone. A man develops a tremendous bond to the hospital in which his life has been saved, and to the surgeon who operated on him. Larry McMurtry, author of *Lonesome Dove* and a friend for over twenty-five years, had had heart bypass surgery done at Johns Hopkins, and made me solemnly promise that I would at least go there for a second opinion. I was, he urged, not even to *consider* having surgery elsewhere—Johns Hopkins was simply the best hospital in the United States, and that was that.

Seymour's message was the same, although delivered with the forcefulness of a natural-born salesman and a true believer—he could not have pushed his own stock with more genuine enthusiasm.

He had never felt better in his life, he told me. His PSA was down to zero point something, virtually zip, just as Pat Walsh had promised. As for the operation, it had been easy, no sweat at all. He had had virtually no pain, the nurses had been terrific, and he was back home in under a week, free of cancer, *cured,* all of which he attributed to the fact that Walsh was a genius—more than a genius, really, a kind of secular saint.

He himself, Seymour confessed to me modestly across the lunch table, was not easily awed. He had made his fortune—by no means an inconsiderable one—early in life, he walked with kings nor lost the common touch, he had advised presidents and been offered ambassadorships; he didn't care about any of that shit, but he knew greatness when he saw it, and when it came to Dr. Walsh he knew himself to be in the presence of a superior man, not only a great scientist but a *caring* physician and a warm and wonderful human being. Dr. Walsh, he told me intently, had *invented* the modern nerve-sparing radical prostatectomy, discovered how to remove the prostate without cutting the nerves that controlled erection, and performed the operation over 1,600 times.

So in awe of the good doctor was Seymour that he had become a major force in the Friends of Pat Walsh, the membership of which consisted, he explained, of Pat Walsh's grateful patients, who were happy—indeed, *honored*—to contribute what they could toward prostate-cancer research at Johns Hopkins.

I was impressed. Here was a man who had been through surgery and emerged from it worshiping his surgeon. Of course, this was the reason for the luncheon, I understood *that*—there was no other reason for Seymour to leave his busy desk to have lunch with a total stranger, as he made it perfectly clear—but his intensity on the subject of prostate cancer was alarming. Not only did he have no small talk, he had no *large* talk. Any effort on my part to change the subject was brushed aside with a wave of his large, well-manicured hand.

Later, I was to understand all too well that cancer, once you have it, is an obsessive subject. The disease literally fills your world to the exclusion of everything else. Cancer is not only the center of the cancer patient's attention—it also puts the patient, for a time, at the center of everybody *else's* attention. Heady stuff.

Before too long I would find that at the drop of a hat I would talk to anybody—friends, casual acquaintances, colleagues, garage attendants, people I hadn't spoken to in years, even total strangers—about my cancer, often in intimate detail that must have made them very uncomfortable indeed. Partly, this is a way of letting off steam, of blunting the fear by sharing the experience with others—not a bad thing at heart. And partly, having cancer is simply the most consuming experience of a lifetime, one that requires the patient's *total* focus and attention. For a time, nothing else seems even remotely as interesting or important as what is going on inside one's body.

Seymour was still at that stage. I would soon find myself doing the same thing, not even *noticing* I was doing it, until several months after my operation Margaret took me to one side after a dinner party and whispered, "You've *got* to stop it!"

I knew exactly what she meant the moment she said it, but there was, apparently, nobody in Seymour's life who wielded that kind of authority over him.

"You'll bounce back from the surgery in no time," he promised me, his eyes glittering with enthusiasm. "I'll give you a piece of advice you'll thank me for. Do what I did. Rent a house in Florida or the islands, go down there for a month or two. Forget about the office. Don't take any calls. Sit in the sun, swim, smell the roses . . ."

How long would it be, I asked, before I could expect to stop smelling the roses and get back to work?

Seymour frowned. No time at all, if that was what I wanted to do, he said. But the thing was to give the body a chance to heal, not to rush it. He punctuated his advice by pointing a breadstick at me for emphasis.

As it happened, I *wasn't* planning to "rush it," assuming "it" finally happened, but I still wanted to know what Seymour's recovery had actually been *like,* rather than hearing another commercial for the Caribbean. How active had he been after the operation? I asked.

Seymour's eyes darkened. He didn't want to talk about specifics or answer questions, it seemed—what he wanted was for me to shut up and accept his advice: have the operation performed at Johns Hopkins, by Pat Walsh, then go to Florida. Like many CEOs, Seymour gave advice that, however well-meant, had the effect of an order: You *will* do this! Otherwise, his attitude implied, you were just wasting his time. "Active?" he asked. "What do you mean active? I bounced back in no time. So will you."

Well, I was concerned, I said, about how long it would be before I could walk, or drive, or resume work ... practical questions like that. How long had it taken him, exactly?

Seymour put his breadstick down and thought about it for a moment, apparently unwillingly. It did not look as if he were dredging up happy memories. He counted the weeks on his fingers thoughtfully. "Well," he said, "I stayed home for about three weeks or a month—until the catheter was removed, you know. . . . Then I went down to Florida. . . ." He closed his eyes for a moment. "You know, the first couple of weeks I was down there, I'd get up from the breakfast table and shuffle over to the pool, maybe fifty yards." He paused. "Then, I'd sit there with *The New York Times* in my lap and cry," he said quietly.

We sat in silence for a few moments, while coffee was served. I sensed that I had heard the truth at last.

"Eventually it got better," Seymour added.

Anything that could make a person as ebullient as Seymour cry over his *New York Times* had to be pretty awful, I thought—and that's without even *asking* what three weeks or a month with a catheter was like. If that was what was in store, it clearly wasn't going to be a picnic.

Seymour sipped at his coffee. "A month or two later, though, I was swimming, playing a little golf, and so on. . . ." He seemed to be trying to cheer himself up. "By the time I got back to the office, I was tanned, fit, and raring to go. . . . Lost twenty pounds, too. I guess you could say the surgery was a blessing in disguise."

It seemed to me that the blessing must have been very well disguised indeed. I looked more closely at Seymour. He was probably telling the truth about losing weight, I thought—his suit looked a size or two larger than he needed—but it didn't look like *healthy* weight loss. There was a hollowness beneath his eyes, a gauntness, which spoke more of pain and suffering than of eating cottage cheese and fresh fruit beneath the Florida sky. His enthusiasm seemed gone now. He looked tired and edgy.

I said that we ought to be getting back to our offices, but he wasn't in any hurry. He ordered another cup of coffee and stirred it slowly, obviously working his way up to something. Now that I had inadvertently deflated his enthusiasm about prostate surgery, he was apparently determined to let it all hang out. "I never had too much of a problem with incontinence," he said. "Some guys do, but I didn't. It lasted a month or so, maybe two, then it got better. No big deal. I'm fine now, except when I laugh hard, then I sometimes wet my pants a bit, but what the hell, who knows, who cares? Big deal! Anyway, in my business, how often do I get to laugh hard?"

"What about sex?"

"Sex? Funny you should ask that. This is kind of a red-letter day, as a matter of fact." It transpired that the night before, Seymour and his wife had made love for the first time since his surgery, about a year before. Sex, he told me, leaning over confidentially, was important to them both, a real factor in their marriage.

I nodded to show that we were on the same wavelength when it came to marital sex.

"My wife is a very passionate woman," he confided. "This whole thing has been very hard on her. She's been a terrific sport about it, but you know how it is. . . . And it's been tough on me, as you can imagine. . . . A year without sex . . . Well, it wasn't easy."

That seemed to me an understatement. I couldn't imagine a year without sex, or even a *month* without sex, come to that. Doctors, I was to discover, were apt to put it as an either-or choice, as in the question "Which would you rather be, sexually potent or alive?" But sexual potency seemed integral to me, one of the joys that made life worth living, and going without it for a year—possibly forever, if Dr. Rous's statistics were to be believed—seemed like a pretty grim prospect. Was sexual potency worth dying for? I didn't think so, but then I hadn't been presented with the choice yet. Seymour was evidently waiting for a comment. "How was it, after all that time?" I asked.

He grinned. "Just great," he said. "I feel alive again, that's how good it was." He waved the waiter away and looked warily to either side to make sure nobody was listening. His voice dropped to a low, gravelly growl. "Of course, you don't get a *full* erection at this stage," he said. "My New York urologist, the guy who took out the catheter, he told me, 'It won't be like it was when you were seventeen, *bubbe,* but with any luck you'll have a *stuffable* erection, if you know what I mean.' " Seymour laughed—not too hard, I noticed.

I didn't think an answer was called for. In any case, I could tell, Seymour was already beginning to regret having opened up to me. Men don't talk to each other about sex—rarely truthfully, at any rate—and Seymour had the look of a man who already wished he had kept his mouth shut. We fought each other for the check—Seymour with a real desire to win, perhaps because he was determined not to be in my debt, now that I knew his secret—and made our good-byes on Fifty-second Street, exchanging cards and promising to keep in touch, to have lunch, dinner, drinks soon, both of us knowing it wouldn't happen.

Seymour turned eastward toward his office. Then, just before he was out of range, he turned back and shouted, "Don't worry, I'll put in a good word for you with Pat Walsh."

8

A FEW DAYS LATER, MARGARET AND I SAW DR. RUSSO FOR MY CON-sultation. Russo clipped my X rays onto the light box on the wall, grimaced at them, and said, "You're a lucky man."

"Lucky?"

"You bet. We caught it just in time. That's good luck in my book."

I decided it was good luck in mine, too.

⁓

MARGARET AND I had been shown into Dr. Russo's office by the ever-cheerful Kathy, and we waited briefly (and nervously) for his arrival.

Russo's office at the Memorial Sloan-Kettering Prostate Cancer Detection Center was light, airy, and blandly impersonal—so impersonal that I came to the conclusion it was not really his. Except for
the bound annals of various urological societies in the bookshelves,
there was nothing at all to connect him with it. There was not even
a desk—just a round table in the center of the room with a pad of
paper in the exact center. I prowled around trying to keep myself
busy, while Margaret leaned against the wall, staring at the plants on
the windowsill through her dark glasses. Neither of us wanted to sit
down.

I had gone out of my way to treat this entire experience as if it
were somehow *normal,* just another activity in town for us to share.
Last week, lunch at a coffee shop on First Avenue and a day of CAT
scans and bone X rays; today, lunch at a strange restaurant I didn't
even know *existed,* on the ground floor of the Barbizon Hotel for
Women, after which we walked over to Dr. Russo's building hand in
hand for my consultation, as if I had taken the afternoon off so we
could see a movie together.

One of the curious things, so far, about my disease was that it had
brought the two of us closer together, almost immediately—as close
as we had been years before, when we were first in love. How often
do married people, after all, spend the afternoon together in midtown Manhattan? In normal circumstances, I would have been at
work in the office and Margaret at home in the country.

I could tell what a strain she was under, so I went over and took
her hand. Just then the door opened and Dr. Russo bustled in, a
manila file folder under one arm.

He fastened my bone X rays up on the wall-mounted light box
and admired them. "Nice work," he said, then asked us to sit down.
He took a chair and indicated the ones on either side of him, so we
sat like the Three Bears, with Dr. Russo as Papa Bear in the center.

I had forgotten how intense Russo was, in his starched white coat,
though it should have been firmly implanted in my mind from that
moment I mentioned earlier, when he put his arm around my shoul-

der and told me that had I been his own *brother*, he could not have urged me more strongly to have a biopsy. *His* day, I thought, must have started at some ungodly hour of the morning—he had probably completed a couple of radical prostatectomies while we were ordering our lunch—but he showed no sign of fatigue beyond dark circles under his eyes. I stared at his hands. They were small, neat, blunt-fingered, *practical* hands, more like a skilled craftsman's than, say, a concert pianist's, hands just right, I decided, for a surgeon. I thought of them probing around deep in my pelvic area with a scalpel, and decided that was something to put out of my mind.

He opened his file and reviewed the results with us—we had heard some of them before, in an abbreviated form, but they had been overshadowed by the good news that the cancer hadn't spread to the bone. Now we were getting down to the nitty-gritty of what I *did* have, not what I didn't.

I had adenocarcinoma, Dr. Russo said. ("Cancer," I whispered to Margaret, who has a certain distrust, typically English, of medical vocabulary.) Russo had a deep voice, and good delivery, like an actor's. He sounded cheerful, although I put this down not to heartlessness but to the fact that the biopsies had proved his initial suspicion correct.

The tumors were deep in the middle left lobe of the prostate, Russo said. That explained why they were hard to find (was I imagining it, or was he suggesting that a deeper biopsy might have located them eighteen months ago?) and might also explain some of my urinary problems, since they were probably pressing on my urethra.

I wondered if they had been missed last time by my urologist— almost certainly so, I thought, judging by the expression on Russo's face. That possibility would continue to haunt and anger Margaret, and still does. As for me, I was still at the very early stages of my experience with cancer, but if there was one thing I had already learned it was that every day you had to start from where you were *at that moment.* Looking backward and thinking about what *might* have been done, or *should* have been done, was a waste of emotional energy.

Besides, in the final analysis, we are all responsible for our own well-being, however tempting it is to blame our misfortunes on doctors. I *should* have been, at my age, more aware of the dangers of prostate cancer, more concerned when I learned that my PSA was 15, instead of waiting eighteen months for it to go up to 22.

I had taken personal responsibility for my cardiovascular fitness, but such was my fear of cancer that I had simply abdicated any responsibility whatsoever the moment the subject came up. Why hadn't I bought the books and started reading about prostate cancer eighteen months before, I asked myself, and made myself a nuisance with questions? I had done nothing of the kind. Cancer is the Big One, and facing the mere *possibility* of it, I simply went on autopilot and put my fate in the hands of my doctors unquestioningly—something I would not have done if the problem had been a torn rotator cuff, or a disk injury, or some irregularity of the heart. Nor was I alone. In this age of fitness consciousness, every man *knows* he has to think about his heart and take responsibility for its well-being; about cancer, he doesn't want to think at all, not just out of fear, but perhaps also because there's no set of routines you can follow that will stave it off. You can't sweat it off, or swim it off, or prevent it by getting on a treadmill every day.

Russo pulled the pad of paper close to him and sketched out a doughnut-shaped object. He divided it into four segments, then drew a narrow tube down the middle. Within one segment he drew two small blobs, each about the size of a peanut, and filled them in. These were the tumors, he said. He extended them until they reached the surface of the prostate. This, he said, is what we are trying to avoid. So long as the tumors are contained in the prostate, we have a situation we can control. Once they break through to the surface, the cancer can spread elsewhere, to the surrounding tissue, to the lymph nodes, and from there through the body.

I was at exactly the stage where a radical prostatectomy was clearly indicated. The procedure was straightforward. He drew the bladder, like a small balloon attached to the top of the urethra. He would cut the prostate free from the bladder, remove it, and suture the bottom of the bladder to the lower portion of the urethra, like so. In a neat, free hand, he showed where the cuts would be made. There were no complications to be expected. There would very likely be some temporary incontinence, but most patients regained continence in time, and where they did not, there were things he could do later on. He did not say what they were, and I did not ask. I would cross that bridge, I decided, when I got to it, God forbid.

What about sex? I asked. Would I be impotent?

Russo gave me a reassuring smile—I supposed it was probably the question he was asked most often. That was hard to answer, he said, though he always kept the patient's quality of life firmly in mind. Two bundles of nerves controlled my ability to have an erection, both of them running across the surface of the prostate. He would shave them free and preserve them, if possible. In most cases where the nerve bundles were preserved, the patient recovered potency eventually. He saw no reason to believe that would not be my case, but of course there was no guarantee.

How long would the operation take?

Between three and four hours, Russo said. I would have a full general anesthetic, and could expect to be in the hospital for five to six days at least.

We sat in silence for a few moments while I digested this information. None of it was very different from what I had read in Dr. Rous's book, but it was one thing to read it and another to hear it addressed to oneself. I was beginning to understand why Rous referred to a radical prostatectomy as a "formidable" operation—not a word to take lightly, coming from a surgeon.

What were my alternatives? I asked. Or was surgery the only option?

Russo admitted that as a surgeon he had a bias in favor of surgery, but, in fact, he did not think there was any alternative. Some men in my condition opted for radiation, and though he was not personally convinced it was the best way to go, there were patients who did well on it. Then, too, some patients were not in physical condition that would permit surgery, so radiation was their only option. Others feared surgery, and chose radiation instead, although, in his opinion, the aftereffects were at least as severe as those of surgery. . . . Radiation would not be his first choice, nor did he think it ought to be mine, but he usually insisted that his patients consult with a radiologist before making up their minds, just so they could hear both sides of the story. Memorial had perhaps the most advanced and sophisticated radiology department in the world, and they were very proud of it.

I had been hoping without conviction that Russo might suggest "watchful waiting," not that mine was a temperament particularly well-suited to waiting of any kind, watchful or not.

What was my Gleason score? I asked.

———

FOR A PATIENT with prostate cancer, knowing his Gleason score is as important as knowing his PSA. As I had learned from reading William Martin's *My Prostate and Me* and Dr. Rous's *The Prostate Book,* the Gleason score indicates both the size and the potential danger of prostate cancers. The oldest and the simplest of the various methods by which pathologists classify prostate cancers, it divides tumors into five grades in ascending order of severity. Grade 1 tumors are small and "well differentiated"—that is, they are distinct from the tissue surrounding them. As they get larger and more "poorly differentiated"—that is, spreading into the tissue surrounding them—they are more serious. A grade 5 tumor may actually have taken over most of the prostate, destroying the healthy tissue.

Confusingly, the Gleason *score* is reached by adding together the two most common grades found in the tissue samples from a biopsy, on a scale ranging from 2 through 10. Thus, a sample with a Gleason *grade* of 3 and another sample with a Gleason *grade* of 2 would equal a Gleason *score* of 5, more or less in the mid-range. A Gleason score from 2 through 4 would indicate small and well-differentiated tumors, perhaps calling for "watchful waiting," while a Gleason score from 8 through 10 might mean that it was already too late to perform a radical prostatectomy. Those, of course, would represent the extremes at both ends of the scale. The vast majority of patients were in the middle, with a Gleason score ranging from 5 through 7.

There are other more sophisticated and refined methods of classifying (or "staging") prostate tumors, more recent than the Gleason system. The Whitmore-Jewett system divides tumors into four stages, A, B, C, and D, then further subdivides each stage to indicate not only the size but the estimated malignancy of the tumor. The TNM system (tumor, node, metastasis) indicates even more precisely the size, the malignancy, and the position of prostate tumors. In all these systems, there is a difference between the value assigned to a tumor on biopsy and that which will be determined by a pathologist once the tumor has been removed and can be physically measured— all too often, the cancer turns out to be worse than was thought.*

The Gleason system was a blunt instrument compared to the Whitmore-Jewett system and the TNM system, but it was at least comparatively easy for a layman to understand. I recalled reading in Professor Martin's book that he had been startled to hear that *his* Gleason score was 7—he had anticipated that it would be 3 or 4. After the surgery his surgeon had told him that it had been "a bad actor," about 2.5 centimeters across, and would probably have reached the surface of the prostate in another year and started to spread through the body. I had assumed my own score would be in the 3-to-4 range myself, since everybody had said that my cancer had been discovered at an early stage and was probably pretty well differentiated. I did not, therefore, think I had heard Russo correctly when he said, "Six."

"Six?"

---

* I am indebted to William Martin for much of this explanation of staging systems. For even more details the reader may care to consult Dr. Rous's book, or *Choices: Realistic Alternatives in Cancer Treatment,* by Marion Morra and Eve Potts, which is a gold mine of helpful information in concise form.

He nodded. I should not be concerned by that. Most patients fell into that range.

A Gleason score of 6 was not something to fool around with, I understood that much: if the books I had read were to be believed, watchful waiting was out of the question. Six placed me close to Martin, and right at the spot Dr. Larrian Marie Gillespie of the Pelvic Pain Center in Beverly Hills calls "the decision from Hell." If I decided to delay, or do nothing, I was playing Russian roulette. (Actually, as Professor Martin points out, the odds in Russian roulette are slightly better, a one-in-six chance of dying, or 16.7 percent, as opposed to an 18 percent* chance of dying, as in my case, not to speak of the fact that a bullet would be merciful compared to what one writer called "a death of rare awfulness.")

If I decided to have the operation, I risked spending the rest of my life with some degree of incontinence and perhaps with total impotence. And that was without considering the possibility of other consequences. I could undergo the surgery and still experience a recurrence of the cancer, in which case I might be incontinent, impotent, *and* a cancer patient for what remained of my life. Or I might spend the rest of my life incontinent, impotent, and wondering whether the surgery was really necessary—whether I might have had ten, or fifteen, or twenty "good" years left to me if I had simply elected to leave well enough alone.

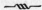

I HAD DRAWN up a list of questions to ask Dr. Russo, but most of them now seemed pointless. He had told me what I needed to know—or, perhaps more accurately, what I had not wanted to know—and now it was up to me.

He broke the silence himself. Numbers didn't mean all that much, he said. I had a dangerous cancer, and I was going to have to have it

* Martin points out that his figure is possibly too high, and was later scaled down somewhat. Still, the comparison he makes is valid, if only as a way of putting the statistical side of prostate cancer in readily understandable perspective.

dealt with. Now was the time to act. There was a very good chance, he thought, that the cancer had not yet reached the surface of the prostate. He would urge me not to delay. He could fit me into his schedule in about four weeks' time—it would take four weeks anyway for me to give enough of my own blood in case it was needed for transfusion purposes, since I could only give one pint a week.

Despite the warmth of the room, I felt a certain chill settle in my bones. I had understood that the cancer *hadn't* reached the surface of the prostate. Was there a chance that it actually already *had*?

Russo shrugged. There was always that chance, he said. One could not rule out surprises. He very much doubted that it would prove to be the case, but the possibility was another good reason to have the surgery done as quickly as possible. One further, but important, advantage of surgery over radiotherapy, he pointed out, was that once the prostate was removed you had all the answers. With radiation, you never knew what was there, or whether the treatment had killed it entirely. He thought it was better to know.

There was one refinement to think about, Russo said. Memorial was involved in an experimental program in which patients with prostate cancer in my range were put on hormones for six months, *then* underwent surgery. The advantage was that the hormone therapy seemed to shrink the tumors, making the surgery easier and more effective. If I liked, he could fit me into this program.

I could tell that Russo was eager for me to agree—it was presumably his program—but I looked at Margaret and shook my head. No doubt if the time ever came when I *had* to have hormone therapy, I would resign myself to it, but in the meantime, once I had made up my mind to have surgery, the sooner it was over and done with, the better. Waiting around, I explained apologetically, just wasn't my style.

Russo took it cheerfully enough. I don't think he had supposed I would agree.

"What about a second opinion?" I asked, feeling a certain embarrassment. I *liked* Russo, I was very confident that he would do a good job, and I didn't want him to feel that I didn't trust him. Still, every-

body had told me to ask for a second opinion, and I felt obliged
to do so.

Russo didn't seem upset. I was perfectly entitled to get a second
opinion, he said. Did I have anyone in mind?

I told him that I was thinking of Dr. Walsh, at Johns Hopkins.

He knew Dr. Walsh, of course, Russo said—they had been together at a recent urological meeting. He was a great surgeon and a
distinguished scientist, no doubt about it.

"I gather he invented the nerve-sparing radical prostatectomy," I
said.

Russo nodded. Yes, Dr. Walsh had invented the procedure, but by
now a lot of surgeons performed it, including Russo himself. In fact,
he liked to think that at Memorial they did about as good an operation as you could have anywhere in the world. Of course, Walsh got
a lot of publicity, but it was a mistake to choose a surgeon by his
celebrity status. I should keep in mind, Russo pointed out, that
Walsh performed only one operation, the nerve-sparing radical
prostatectomy.

Russo, on the other hand, as he made clear, did all sorts of operations—why, just the other day he had given a patient an artificial
bladder, groundbreaking surgery. Which was better? he wondered
aloud. A surgeon who performed the same operation over and over
again, or a surgeon whose skills were constantly being challenged?

It was a rhetorical question, since Russo was still talking, more intense than ever. I should understand that sparing the nerve bundles
was not the be-all and end-all it was made out to be. People made a
big fuss about it, but it wasn't the whole story by a long shot. Sparing the nerve bundles was all very well—and he was as good at sparing them as anyone, if he did say so himself, *when they could be
spared*—but I should consider this: the purpose of the operation was
to remove the cancer.

Memorial was a cancer hospital, and cancer was the enemy, it was
as simple as that. He would give me the best operation he could, and
it was pretty damn good, but he would always err on the side of

safety, removing as much tissue as he felt he had to. There was no point in saving the nerve bundles at the risk of leaving behind cancerous tissue, even if it was only a microscopic amount. I should bear in mind that a microscopic amount could eventually kill the patient. Surgery was a macroscopic solution to a microscopic problem. One cell could kill you, if it made its way to the lymph nodes. If *he* operated on me, Russo said, he would do everything possible to save my sexuality, but not at the possible expense of my life.

That made sense to me, much as it wasn't something I wanted to hear. Did he think that he would be able to spare my nerve bundles?

There was no way to know that until the surgery, he said. Once the surgery was under way, everything would be clear. It was his practice, for example, to remove the pelvic lymph nodes for dissection and an immediate pathological examination before continuing the operation. If they were clear, fine. If they were *not,* he would not continue with the operation.

I let this sink in. Obviously, if the pelvic lymph nodes showed signs of cancer, there was no point in putting the patient through the rigors of major surgery. Once the cancer spread to the lymph nodes, there was no cure—it was more humane to sew the patient back up and put him on palliative therapy to preserve his "quality of life" for as long as possible.

On this note Russo closed. The decision was mine. I should let him know as soon as possible.

We stood and shook hands, then he led us out to the waiting room, where he was joined by Kathy and Dr. Fleishner, who had performed my biopsy ten days before—already it seemed like a lifetime. They stood together in a small, photogenic group, Memorial Sloan-Kettering's prostate-cancer A-team, smiling as if I were the prodigal son. I felt, obscurely, a profound loyalty to them, as if we had been through a war together. I liked them, trusted them, would be perfectly content, here and now, to leave my fate in their hands.

I wanted to turn around and walk back to Russo and tell him I didn't need a second opinion, not from a radiologist, not from Pat

Walsh, that he was my man, but something, perhaps a certain caution, perhaps also the notion of having to explain to all those well-meaning friends, acquaintances, and total strangers that I hadn't given their advice to seek a second opinion from Walsh any thought at all, prevented me from doing it.

I pressed the elevator button instead. At bottom, I thought, this was the most important decision of my life. I owed it to myself to get a second opinion before I made up my mind, even if it went against my grain to do so.

—⁂—

DOWN ON THE street, in the late-afternoon sunshine, Margaret took my hand and squeezed it. "You're going to see Walsh, aren't you?" she asked.

"I think so," I said. "I think I have to." I knew she didn't want me to. I could tell that she liked Russo (as I did). And I could guess that she didn't want to drag this experience out, that her own nerves were already at the breaking point. Besides, if I was going to have the operation—and that was as good as decided, unless the radiologist produced a rabbit out of his hat at the last moment—it would be much easier to do it in New York than in Baltimore. Margaret could stay in the apartment, as opposed to camping out in a strange city in a hotel.

We crossed Lexington Avenue and walked slowly east, hand in hand. Rush hour was building up, and people hurried past us while we seemed to have all the time in the world, casual strollers.

It was an illusion, of course; time was already pressing down on us, in the shape of irrevocable decisions that had to be made quickly and that would have seemed unthinkable only ten days ago. The truth was that having cancer was a world of its own, like living in a kind of cocoon; it made everything outside seem unreal and unimportant—appointments, obligations, rush hour, work, none of that seemed to matter or have any real significance compared to what was going on in the lower left lobe of my prostate, silently and painlessly at this very moment.

"You mustn't let people push you into choosing Dr. Walsh," Margaret said.

"I'm not. What gave you that idea?"

"I know you."

I was silent.

"I just want you to make up your own mind, that's all," Margaret said. "Don't listen to other people."

"I'm not, I promise," I said, though I wondered if that was really true. "But I *do* want to see Walsh first—*if* we can get an appointment with him reasonably soon. I like Russo, but there's too much at stake here to take one doctor's word for what has to be done, however much I like him."

Margaret squeezed my hand again, harder this time. "Don't worry so much about the sex," she whispered to me. "I'd rather have you alive."

I thought it over, and decided it was the nicest thing she'd ever said to me.

9

THERE MAY BE MORE CHILLING PLACES IN A HOSPITAL THAN THE RAdiology department, but not many. Memorial Sloan-Kettering's is no exception. Here, there is no escaping the reality of cancer and what it does to people—what it could do to *me*, I couldn't help thinking. Cancer patients waited, slumped in wheelchairs, for their treatments or for someone to wheel them back up to their rooms. Some of them seemed to have been waiting endlessly, but I couldn't help noticing that none of them had brought any reading material. Since I'm the kind of person who can't endure a wait of two or three minutes without something to read—I move everywhere with a briefcase containing at least a couple of manuscripts, a book, *The New York Times,* the latest magazines, and a folder of correspondence to answer—I found this spectacle chilling. These people were so exhausted, or perhaps merely so wrapped up in the struggle to survive, that they were beyond reading. Some of them waited hours without betraying the smallest sign of boredom or curiosity, eyes half closed, breathing slowly, as if they were doing yoga, except they weren't. I tried to imagine myself in a similar position, and couldn't.

Fortunately, I had come prepared, and had urged Margaret to do the same. I write "fortunately" because I soon realized how important it was to keep Margaret's mind off the silent, uncomplaining figures in the wheelchairs, and also because the radiologist, unlike Dr. Russo, was a man whose specialty required him to do several things at the same time. He didn't even *have* an office, or at any rate not one we were shown to. Here life-and-death decisions were being made all the time—the entire staff was on the move, in action. One of the nurse's aides put us in an examination room and left us there with the door open, in a perfect position to observe the radiology department at work and, as it turned out, with ample time to do so. From time to time, bulletins were brought to us: "The doctor is on his way"; or, sometime later, "The doctor has been delayed"; or, least promising of all, "Don't worry, the doctor hasn't forgotten about you."

On a couple of occasions we actually *saw* the doctor himself, rushing godlike (I am thinking of Mercury with the winged feet) past his patients, followed by a flying wedge of interns, assistants, aides, and nurses, most of them holding out charts for him to sign. He was a tall, athletic-looking man, clad in a green scrub suit, who looked like a general in command. I had brought a manuscript to edit, while Margaret did the *Times* crossword. From time to time I wandered into the adjacent hallway (we had been *forbidden* to leave our examination room for fear we wouldn't be there when the doctor did actually appear) to call my office and report that I would be late. Eventually, there seemed no point to doing that: enough of the day had gone by to make my return to the office doubtful.

When he turned up at last, the radiologist moved Margaret out of the room so he could do a quick DRE (another quick slap of the latex glove), then called her back in. He was, on closer examination, a bigger man than I had thought, muscular and intense, with the kind of forceful personality that filled the tiny room. We sat on small plastic chairs, while the doctor towered over us, leaning against the examination couch. Now that he was finally with us, he gave us his full attention. Assistants and nurses kept appearing with questions and problems, but he waved them away. The door remained open, however, which gave me the surreal impression that my consultation was being observed, if not actually overheard, by everybody on the floor. The doctor leaned forward—the three of us were jammed in close together, knee to knee, like old friends in a cocktail-bar booth—and smiled. "I felt a little bump or ridge on the prostate," he said. "I guess everybody has told you about that."

That caught my attention. Not only had nobody told me about that, my internist had even specifically said that he *couldn't* feel anything. I shook my head.

He shrugged. "Well, *I* did," he said cheerfully. "Harder than the surrounding tissue. Of course, it *could* be scar tissue from the biopsies. You never know. . . ."

"Or?" I asked.

"Or the cancer may have reached the surface of the prostate. It's always a possibility."

"Wouldn't it have shown up on the ultrasound or the CAT scan?"

"Maybe. Usually. Listen, even if it *has* reached the surface, don't worry. There are plenty of things we can do."

His style was bluff heartiness, coupled with a certain no-nonsense, take-it-or-leave-it forcefulness and a lot of aggressive body language to match. He aimed it more at Margaret than at me, perhaps because she is an extremely beautiful woman. If so, he'd made a mistake. Several hours of waiting in the radiology department had strained Margaret's composure to the breaking point. She is not a squeamish woman—she had been through hell during her father's death in an English country hospital, and toughed it out during her mother's descent into senility in a nursing home—but the ghost figures in wheelchairs outside the open door represented everything she feared for me, and doubtless for herself—some combination of disease and helplessness that was her worst nightmare.

In the meantime, I was still struggling with the idea that my cancer might already have reached beyond the prostate capsule. I asked him whether he really thought that was possible with a Gleason 6 tumor and a PSA of 22. "Sure," he said affably, "no question about it."

If that were the case, I asked, what were the odds that it had spread? He looked thoughtful. "About fifty-fifty," he said.

He said it loud and clear, as if he weren't sure that Margaret was paying attention. Then, just in case she had missed the point, he said, "Say, one in two."

He looked at Margaret as though expecting her to say something, but she was silent. I could see tears running down her cheeks from under her impenetrable sunglasses. For the first time since I had been diagnosed with prostate cancer, she was crying. I touched her hand, but it didn't do any good. It was as if the radiologist had inadvertently breached her defenses, determined to make the reality of the thing sink in. I wondered aloud if she wanted to leave the room and walk a bit in the corridor, but she shook her head, giving me a glance I interpreted as "Let's get this over with."

Now that the doctor had our attention, though, he was in no hurry. He set out on a leisurely description of the history of radiation, pausing from time to time to make sure that we were listening and understood.

Margaret stared into the middle space, tears still running down her cheeks uncontrollably, sobbing gently but noticeably while the doctor talked on enthusiastically and oblivious. He explained that the traditional method of radiation used in cases of prostate cancer was external beam radiation, in which a powerful beam was aimed precisely at the site of the tumor and repeated at frequent intervals over a period of time until the cancer was killed—usually four to five times a week for a period of six to seven weeks. He himself, he said, was constantly amazed at how well patients did while undergoing the treatment. He had patients who put on their running clothes and jogged across the Park from their apartments to Memorial in the early morning for their treatment, jogged home afterward, then changed and went to their offices to put in a full day's work. When you compared that to surgery, where the patient undergoes an extremely invasive procedure, spends a week in the hospital, then eight to twelve weeks of recuperation, plus all the debilitating possibilities . . . He threw his arms up in the air. Well, there simply *was* no comparison, was there?

I sensed that an answer was called for (and was not going to come from Margaret, who was still crying); besides, I had to admit that the radiologist's spiel was persuasive, despite the doubts of Drs. Rous and Russo on the subject of radiation. I imagined myself jogging across the Park, having my treatment, picking up my *Times* and a croissant on the way home, then going off to the office. . . . It sounded a lot better than anything I had heard about surgery from those who had had it. Were there any side effects? I asked. Dr. Rous, in his book, had mentioned a few, including loss of bowel control, and even permanent rectal damage. The radiologist waved away these problems impatiently. They did happen, he admitted, but not frequently, and there were plenty of things that could be done to help the patient.

What if the radiation didn't work? I wanted to know. Was it still possible to have surgery? He was cautious, for the first time. It was certainly *possible*, yes, but rarely successful. Due to the inevitable damage radiation did to the surrounding tissue, there wasn't much a surgeon could do after the fact. Such procedures were known as "salvage operations," which pretty much said it all. In the event that radiation failed, hormone therapy was usually the next step, perhaps accompanied by a bilateral orchiectomy.

I raised an eyebrow.

The surgical removal of both testicles, he explained, the object being to eliminate the body's production of testosterone, without which the prostate cancer couldn't grow. Really, there wasn't much difference between an orchiectomy and hormone therapy. The latter was chemical castration; the former, surgical castration, that's all. He gave Margaret a smile. It's not nearly as bad as it sounds, he reassured her.

By now, however, Margaret was beyond the capacity for reply, sunk into a kind of dumb misery as the doctor continued relentlessly, determined to make her understand what she didn't even want to *hear*. It wasn't any one thing that had put her over the edge—it was the big picture he was painting, the unspeakable horrors that might lie before us and that we hadn't even considered. Dr. Russo's had been the light touch: we've caught it early on and I can take care of it. He had left the downside unspoken, a delicately suspended sword of Damocles. The radiologist's view was darker. To give him credit, I do not think he wanted to frighten us—he simply seemed to feel that we should know just how bad it could get. Surgeons, he implied, offer the patients a simple fix for a complicated problem. They tell you what you want to hear, not the whole truth, which is that there *is* no simple fix—prostate cancer, like any other kind of cancer, is a moving picture, not a still picture. The cancer grows, moves, mutates, shrinks, recurs; clinical tests can only show you what its status is *today, now,* not predict what it will be tomorrow, or five years from now. The radiologist even had charts and papers to give us for further reading. He stabbed at the statistics with a blunt finger. Even if the cancer has spread, he told us, radiology offered far better odds for survival than surgery—it was all there in black and white, for us to study at our leisure. A survival rate of five to seven years, even with sky-high PSAs—go find a surgeon who could show you those kinds of results!

I could see that Margaret was taking in only the numbers, assuming that the radiologist was telling us that *my* "survival rate" was five to seven years, whereas he was, in fact, merely outlining an aggressive case for radiology and talking averages. Still, I thought it best to head him off at the pass and turn the consultation more firmly toward my case specifically, before Margaret broke down altogether.

Did he think my case lent itself to radiation? I asked. I had been given the impression that it did not. Was that a mistake?

He explained that external beam radiation did not seem to be a viable option for me. In general, for patients like me, he preferred a second method, radioactive implantations, with which he had had very good results. This method required a brief but essentially painless hospitalization, during which thin tubes, hardly more than needles, were inserted *precisely* into the site of the cancer, and through which tiny radioactive "seeds" were then implanted to destroy the tumor. The exact placing of the needles was crucial to the success of the operation, and this part of the procedure was worked out beforehand on a computer, after which a plastic mold of the appropriate area of the body was made so that the final placement of the seeds would be precise. Once the seeds were implanted, I should understand, they were not removed—it was a one-way street, so to speak. Their potency declined rapidly, and they soon became completely safe. So long as they *were* active, I should discourage children, pregnant women, and perhaps even Margaret from sitting in my lap for a few days—he laughed—but beyond that the radioactivity was not particularly dangerous, and should not be a concern.

His description of the process was fascinating, and presented, I thought, a not unattractive option. A day or two in the hospital, a comparatively noninvasive procedure, and off you go about your normal business while tiny radioactive seeds in your prostate do their work. It sounded a good deal better than surgery, and had a nice, clean, high-tech ring to it.

Were there any aftereffects? I wondered. In the short term, no, he replied. Patients quickly resumed their normal routines, including exercise, and sexual function was not usually impaired.

The idea of an alternative to surgery that *didn't* involve incontinence and impotence was appealing, and I said so. The radiologist agreed, albeit with something less than total enthusiasm. I should understand, he said, that there was no such thing as a free lunch where prostate cancer was concerned. The *long-term* effects of radiation were a concern, both for the external-beam and the implantation methods. In a certain percentage of cases, incontinence and impotence *did,* in fact, set in—six months or so after the procedure. Unfortunately, when that was the case, these conditions were irreversible.

Did I understand him correctly? Was he saying that while I might experience impotence and incontinence immediately after surgery, there was a chance they would diminish or altogether disappear in the months following, whereas with radiation I would feel perfectly normal after the procedure, only to risk becoming permanently incontinent and impotent later on? He nodded encouragingly. That was about the size of it. It didn't happen to *everyone,* of course, but it could happen, and I should be aware of the possibility.

I said that radiation didn't sound all that attractive a proposition, now that he had spelled it out in detail, particularly since if it *didn't* work, there was very little chance that surgery would be a possibility; whereas in the reverse case, radiation could be helpful if the surgery was unsuccessful.

He acknowledged this. Radiation offered many advantages over surgery, he said, but it wasn't the answer for everyone.

What, I asked directly—since the radiologist, to give him his due, seemed less Olympian than Dr. Russo—would *he* do if he were in my position, with a Gleason score of 6 and a PSA of 22?

"I would opt for the surgery," he said firmly. I did not think that this doctor and I were about to become friends for life, but I admired his bluff honesty. Not many specialists will unhesitatingly recommend a rival treatment.

The determining factor, he went on, was that my prostate was considerably enlarged. The larger the prostate, the more radiation was needed to do the job; it was as simple as that. In my case, not only were the tumors inconveniently placed, but the enlarged prostate would require a dose of radioactivity so high that it would inevitably affect the surrounding tissue and organs. It was a pity, but there it was.

Where was I intending to have my surgery performed? he wanted to know. I told him that it looked as though I were going to choose between Dr. Russo, there at Memorial, or Pat Walsh, at Johns Hopkins.

"Ah," he said, "Pat Walsh." Far be it for him to compare surgeons, but I should not underrate Dr. Russo, or Memorial. They did a great job of surgery here, I should have no doubt about that.

I assured him that I didn't, but I felt I wanted a second opinion, from Dr. Walsh. He nodded. He could understand that. Of course.

Finally he showed us out of the examination room, where we seemed to have been sitting for days, and taking Margaret by the arm, he hurried us down the corridor while his staff jogged along behind us, trying to catch his attention. I thought it was not an accident that they all wore running shoes—their chief set a breathless pace, his patterned soles squeaking on the slickly polished linoleum.

He was exuberantly cheerful, like the host of a successful party. I should read up on the statistics, he warned me, before going to see Walsh. Look at his numbers. Compare them to Russo's numbers. Numbers tell the story. Yes, yes, he knew all about the nerve-sparing radical prostatectomy, but that wasn't the whole story, no way. I would see for myself, his own numbers were as good or better than those Walsh had published, if you were talking about five- or ten-year survival. . . .

We had reached the nurses' station now, at the farthest point of his domain. He was pulling papers out of drawers and files behind the nurses' station, shoving them into the copying machine himself. Here was *his* paper; here was Dr. Walsh's latest paper; here were papers from various European studies. . . . He took a yellow fluorescent Hi-Liter and marked off charts, graphs, rows of numbers for us to study. Some of the papers, he did not have time to copy. He lent them to me, extracting the promise that I would return them after I had made copies for myself. He shook hands with both of us heartily, and I had the impression that he was really sorry to see us go. Like most doctors, he seemed to me a true believer in his own specialty, at his happiest when talking about it, but unlike many of them, he was objective about it when push came to shove. If he did not mince words, that too was perhaps a blessing, however heavily disguised. Perhaps nobody else could have made Margaret finally listen to the statistics of survival and absorb them, however unwillingly.

I took her arm, and we walked out of the hospital. She lifted her sunglasses and dabbed at her eyes. "I can't go through that again," she said. "If Baltimore is going to be anything like that, I don't want to go."

"He didn't say anything I haven't already told you."

"I don't care about his numbers," she said fiercely.

"All he was saying is that there's a chance I'll die, in five years, or ten, whatever we do. We *know* that."

"One in two."

"That's only if it's spread. . . . It's nothing like as bad as that if you actually look at the numbers—"

"I hate statistics."

"You can't hate facts."

"Oh yes I can."

"That isn't logical."

"I don't care."

When I got home I put the papers, with their bright yellow fluorescent marks, on the hall table. Late that night I found Margaret reading them in bed.

—✺—

THE TRUTH OF the matter, as we discussed later—and would still be hashing over on our way down to Baltimore—was that the statistics *didn't* tell you much, except that most of Dr. Walsh's patients lived longer than ten years after surgery—but then, so did people who had radiation.

You can read statistics in a lot of different ways, but in the end the one that mattered most—or at least caught my eye most—was a small note in a paper by Dr. Walsh referring to a Swedish study of patients with "small, well-differentiated tumors" in whom "watchful waiting" was undertaken. At ten years, 13 percent of the patients were dead and 50 percent of the patients had experienced "progression of cancer to the bone or adjacent structures." Most patients who experienced this progression died—very unpleasantly, as the study made it clear—within the next five years. Watchful waiting suddenly seemed less attractive.

Admittedly, the average age of the men in the Swedish study was seventy-two, which would seem to me to have argued that most of the men would have died of *something* within the next ten or fifteen years, even if it wasn't cancer, but the message was still clear enough: doing nothing was a potentially fatal mistake, and since the radiologist himself had ruled out radiation, it was going to have to be surgery. It wasn't a question of *what,* but *who,* just as I had expected it would be.

Still, the numbers were so interesting that I began to mark them off myself with my own Hi-Liter. I was struck by a table that indicated the recovery of potency after a radical prostatectomy. Based upon 503 patients at Johns Hopkins, the return of sexual function among men in my age group (sixty to sixty-nine) occurred in 69 percent of the patients when both nerve bundles were preserved intact, in 50 percent when one nerve bundle was "partially excised," and in 47 percent when one nerve bundle was "widely excised." In other words, I thought, *at worst,* even if Dr. Walsh was only able to preserve *one* nerve bundle, there was almost a fifty-fifty chance I would regain potency.

The chart did not mention the possibility of losing *both* nerve bundles, I noticed, but I decided not to dwell on that. I firmly marked that particular passage in yellow Hi-Liter, and told myself that things were perhaps not as bleak as they had seemed in the radiologist's examination room.

In the morning, however, it occurred to me that a one-in-two chance of regaining some measure of sexual potency wasn't really that cheerful a prospect after all. And even if Dr. Walsh succeeded in preserving *both* nerve bundles, there was still one chance in three, more or less, that I would be impotent.

That was the trouble with statistics. What cheered you up when you read it at night, depressed you when you thought about it again in the morning, and vice versa.

I bundled the papers together and put them in my briefcase. I would have to ask Dr. Walsh to interpret them for us himself.

10

WE TOOK THE LAST FLIGHT POSSIBLE DOWN TO BALTIMORE. HAVING checked into the hotel, we ordered crab cakes, the local specialty, from room service and watched a movie, but our mood was not festive.

Margaret was very reasonably concerned about how I would get home from Baltimore after my release from the hospital. With the baffling unhelpfulness so typical of airlines since deregulation, Baltimore had become a difficult place to reach directly. To reach our nearest commercial airport, Stewart International in Newburgh, New York, it would be necessary for us to fly a dog's-leg course from Baltimore to Pittsburgh (in the wrong direction and completely out of our way), change planes there—with a two-hour stopover—then fly on to Newburgh, which was about an hour away from where we lived.

This did not sound like something I would want to be doing a week after major surgery—it wasn't a trip that made all that much sense when you were feeling well, for that matter. An alternative would be to fly from Baltimore to La Guardia, in New York City, then go home by car—a two-hour drive. Would I be up to getting through La Guardia, one of the most crowded, difficult, and permanently unfinished airports in the world, or the two-hour car trip home? Amtrak was another possibility, but how well would I handle several hours on a train, followed by an hour or so in New York City traffic, then two hours more on the parkways north? There was no answering these questions. I simply presumed that if other people had managed, I could, and that if I put one foot in front of another, however slowly, I would eventually get where I wanted to go. Neither of these presumptions convinced Margaret, so I added this to the list of questions I wanted to ask Dr. Walsh.

It should surprise nobody that we spent the evening discussing travel plans for my return from the hospital. This kind of thing is a common reaction to cancer. Trivial problems take on undue importance. There is a natural human tendency to turn molehills into mountains in the face of disaster, if only because thinking about relatively unimportant or pedestrian details gives people the illusion of being in control of their fate. *You* can make decisions, after all, about travel arrangements, or hotel reservations, or which dressing gown you're going to bring with you to the hospital, or whether or not you should go for a TV in your hospital room.

Not, mind you, that travel was my only concern. I was trying to think ahead to the period of time *after* the surgery, perhaps as a way of not thinking about the surgery itself, but nothing in the books or the previous consultations with Dr. Russo and the radiologist had suggested what my life would be like during my recuperation, or what changes, if any, I would have to make at home.

Now that I had—at last—accepted the fact that I was going to have surgery, there were a lot of questions I wanted answered. How much pain would be involved? If I had the operation in Baltimore, who would look after me once I got home? (I could hardly travel back to Baltimore every time I had a pain or a problem!) Would I need nursing care once I was home, and if so, what kind and for how long? Would I be able to manage the steep stairs of our house—it was built in the eighteenth century—or should I plan to remain downstairs during my recuperation? (But there were no bathrooms downstairs, so that wouldn't work out. . . .)

I needed a detailed plan, fully spelled out, not the kind of well-meant generalizations I had been getting from fellow prostate-cancer sufferers like Seymour or, so far, from my doctors. I wanted some-body to be in *charge*—the sooner, the better.

I was in the right mood for our consultation with Patrick Walsh.

—⁓—

JOHNS HOPKINS WAS a world apart from any of the New York hospitals I knew. Its sheer size—it covered several city blocks—was overwhelming, but what really caught the eye was not so much the size but the *scale*—you entered it through vast, modernistic lobbies, with immensely high vaulted ceilings, and traveled from one part to another through gleaming, fluorescent-lit corridors on people movers. It reminded me, vaguely, of my father Vincent Korda's sets for the film of H. G. Wells's *The Shape of Things to Come,* or perhaps Charles de Gaulle Airport, outside Paris. It was as if the architecture were expressly designed to dwarf people. Here and there, there were small attempts at humanizing the place—an outdoor café, of all things—but the overall impression was that of a small, self-contained city, which, in a way, was exactly what it was: a hospital city, rather than the city's hospital.

We had been given exact instructions, plus a map of Johns Hopkins, by Dr. Walsh's staff, so we knew exactly where to go and what to expect. I filled in innumerable forms in the reception area, was issued an orange plastic "credit" card, which I was to keep with me at all times and which would function like the beads that are used instead of money at a Club Med, and waited briefly in line to have a blood sample taken. I have never much liked having blood taken, but I was soon going to get used to it—a small dividend of prostate cancer. Hardly anything happened at Johns Hopkins without a blood sample, it appeared.

We made our way to Dr. Walsh's domain, a cool, gray, elegantly appointed space not unlike the international-departures lounge of a modern airport. Here, too, there was evidence of a precise *method,* a carefully worked out plan—go to this desk, then to that one, fill in this form, then that one, and eventually there you are, seated on a long gray couch under subdued, soothing lighting, waiting your turn.

Everybody we met was polite, knew who we were, and knew exactly where we were going next. Everybody made it clear that here, at any rate, Pat Walsh's word was law; when his staff mentioned his name, and they invoked it often, it was in tones of awe—so much so that although the area was quite crowded, hardly anybody talked above a whisper, so that there was a certain *reverent* quality to the ambience, like that in a cathedral, where even the tourists talk in undertones.

—⁓—

A FEW WORDS about Patrick C. Walsh, M.D. He is—as I discovered from reading *Hopkins Medical News* and *Prostate Cancer Update,* issues of which were spread out everywhere, his photograph splashed on the covers—not only one of Johns Hopkins's star surgeons but urologist-in-chief at the James Buchanan Brady Urological Institute of the Johns Hopkins Medical Institutions, as well as David Hall McConnell Professor and Director of the Department of Urology. He is teacher, surgeon, administrator, his presence unmistakably omnipresent.

We had arrived, despite many complaints from Margaret, ridiculously early. My level of anxiety was such that, left to my own, I would have been at Johns Hopkins at dawn for our ten o'clock appointment. I had the time to read the profile of Dr. Walsh in the *Hopkins Medical News* twice. I was delighted to learn that he had "drastically reduced the operation's worst side effects—impotence and incontinence." Described as "bespectacled [and] soft-spoken" (as well as "the Michelangelo of prostate surgery"), Walsh had been dismayed by the difficulties of prostate surgery, which had not changed much since the operation was first performed, at Johns Hopkins, nearly one hundred years ago. In performing a radical prostatectomy, the surgeon literally operated blind, in large measure because of the enormous loss of blood. "The operation used to be performed in a sea of blood," Dr. Walsh was quoted as saying.

Walsh's first great contribution to prostate surgery was to work out the exact anatomy of the blood vessels surrounding the prostate, and then to invent a way of stanching the flow of blood. With a "blood-less field," it became possible for the surgeon to see what he was doing at last, as a result of which the percentage of patients who were rendered completely incontinent by the surgery dropped dramatically.

His second contribution was equally revolutionary. It had been usual for the surgeon to cut through the two bundles of penile nerves in order to remove the prostate, thus ensuring that the patient would be impotent. These nerves, it was presumed, ran *through* the prostate and therefore could not be saved. Walsh, once he had his "bloodless field," was skeptical of this. In 1981, he spent his forty-third birthday, it appeared, on vacation in Holland, dissecting stillborn infants in the company of a retired Dutch professor of anatomy, and discovered that his skepticism was justified: the penile nerves did *not* run through the prostate but were *outside* it, attached to a membrane.* It must therefore, he decided, be possible to remove the prostate without damaging the nerves, thus preserving sexual function.

I did not know which was the more remarkable—the fact that surgeons had been performing radical prostatectomies for ninety years or so without being able to see what they were doing, and without even knowing the anatomical structure of the area in which they were working, or the fact that Dr. Walsh, if *Hopkins Medical News* was to be believed, had spent his forty-third birthday dissecting stillborn infants.

I read the passage out loud to Margaret, who made a face and said, "I wish you hadn't told me that."

Walsh and his Dutch associate kept studying the anatomy of the prostate until, in 1982, Walsh was able to remove the prostate of a fifty-two-year-old man without damage to the nerve bundles. The lucky patient "regained his sexual function in a year." Walsh had brought about a revolution in the treatment of prostate cancer.

Walsh's colleagues in urology had paid him the ultimate compliment of imitation. Still, it explained, I thought, the strong sense of

---

* It is easier to see the exact anatomy of the prostate in an infant, since it has not yet been covered with an adult layer of fat.

rivalry that seemed to exist between Walsh and other urologists, except perhaps those who had trained under him, of which, by now, there were not a few.

I read on, mesmerized by the article, which I wished I'd read two years before. In a sidebar, I found an explanation for much that had puzzled me about my biopsies. One of Walsh's assistants described the difficulty of securing meaningful tissue samples as "like looking *with* a needle in a haystack."

The thin biopsy needle captures tiny plugs of tissue from the prostate, each no more than a millimeter across, but given the thin, random spread of most prostate cancers, the biopsy can produce a false negative rate of as much as 25 percent.

I wondered if that had been the case with *my* first biopsy, when my PSA had been 15? Was my urologist reading a false negative then? Did it really mean that one out of every four men who came away from his urologist with good news after a biopsy for prostate cancer was, in fact, receiving not only false hope but very dangerously misleading news? Apparently so. It could not have been made clearer that anybody with a high PSA not only ought to seek out the best and most aggressive program for further testing, but also ought to have it done at frequent intervals—certainly once every twelve months, even if the results were negative.

What chilled me, reading the article, was that I hadn't known anything about prostate cancer until I had it. Women were taught how to watch for the early warning signs of breast cancer, and warned about the dangers of complacency, but most men knew next to nothing about the leading type of cancer in men—and the fastest growing, for doctors at Johns Hopkins estimate that by the year 2000 the United States will experience "a 37 percent increase in the yearly number of prostate-cancer deaths, and a whopping 90 percent increase in new cases each year."*

---

* Janet Farrer Worthington, "Outliving Prostate Cancer," *Hopkins Medical News,* Winter 1992.

That was the bad news—grim enough, one would have thought, to alert men to the danger, if the news had been widespread, which it was not. The good news was that in its early stages it is curable.

The article cited the case of Jim Berry, a syndicated cartoonist, who was fifty-eight when he was diagnosed as having prostate cancer after an elevated PSA test—a situation very similar to my own, I thought. Dr. Walsh had performed Berry's radical prostatectomy successfully, giving him, at the end of a year, "a clean bill of health." Berry had been able to work from his bed within a few days after surgery, and ended up with "good" continence and a satisfactory de- gree of potency. "The whole thing was a big success," he said. I couldn't help noticing, however, that at the end of the piece Berry was quoted as saying of his surgery and recuperation: "The whole thing wasn't a walk in the park or anything."

Hopkins Medical News did not go into detail about *that* aspect of Berry's experience. A pity, since it was exactly what I wanted to know.

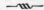

AT THE STROKE of 10:00, one of Dr. Walsh's secretaries ushered us into a small, neatly appointed examination room, where Dr. Walsh himself appeared a moment later. My first impression of him was of his enormous self-confidence, noteworthy even by the standards of surgeons, a notably self-confident bunch, and only slightly disguised by a careful, almost old-fashioned, courtesy. In photographs, Dr. Walsh's slightly protuberant pale-blue eyes had a pixieish quality to them, even from behind the big glasses, as if he were secretly full of high spirits. In real life, though, his eyes—even bluer than in pic- tures—had a certain steely look to them—bright, hard stainless steel, at that. High spirits were not in evidence. Though conspicuously po- lite and soft-spoken, Dr. Walsh was not, I judged, a man to be trifled with—not that I had any intention of trifling with him. Margaret left the room while he performed the ritual DRE, then, when he was done, he sat down at a small built-in desk while she and I sat, knee- to-knee, beside him, as if he were about to receive our confession.

"You must be an important man," he said. "All sorts of people have been calling me about you." He mentioned Ken Aretsky and my CEO acquaintance, Seymour. He shook his head. "I'm impressed." His expression made it obvious that he was more *amused* than impressed.

I had forgotten all about Seymour's promise, made as we parted after that grim lunch, but Seymour clearly had not. I was impressed, even touched. I wondered whether I would have done the same for a stranger—but as I was soon to discover, cancer survivors are never total strangers to each other. There may not be much to say in favor of the disease, but the one thing it *does* do is to create a genuine camaraderie. Survival is a powerful bond.

I told Dr. Walsh that everyone I had spoken to insisted I do nothing until I consulted with him. He gave me a small, self-deprecating smile, and nodded, as if urging me to get on with it. I quickly filled him in on my consultation with Dr. Russo at Memorial Sloan-Kettering. "I gather that you know each other," I added, since there had been no sign of recognition from Dr. Walsh. "Apparently, you saw each other recently at some urological meeting?"

Dr. Walsh's smile was unwavering, but he shook his head. Memorial was a fine hospital, though, he said. I could not go wrong there.

There was a brief silence while I digested this, wishing I had never brought up Russo's name. I wished I could kick myself, in fact. Had I committed, unknowingly, some grave breach of medical etiquette? Had I perhaps misunderstood Dr. Russo? It occurred to me that Dr. Walsh might simply be putting things in perspective: I had come to Johns Hopkins to see *him*, after all, so Dr. Russo's opinions about my case, whatever they might be, were of no consequence, a waste of his time. I decided not to fill him in about my radiological consultation, or my doubts about whether my first biopsy had been performed correctly. Now that I was actually here, in front of the man, my only fear was that he would turn me down as a patient.

Dr. Walsh perused my file silently for a few minutes, then looked up, frowning. I was on the borderline, he said. He did not like enlarged prostates, and mine was considerably enlarged.

My heart sinking, I asked what kind of problems that created.

The surgical problems were not so bad, Dr. Walsh said, though they existed, but I should understand that an enlarged prostate like mine could slow down my recovery of continence very considerably. The bladder had to work harder and harder to force the urine down through the obstructed urethra. Gradually, over time, the bladder became more muscular, and its walls therefore thickened. This had two consequences. The first was that there was simply less *space* left in the bladder for urine, so that the bladder signaled it was full when, in fact, it was only partly full—hence the frequent need to urinate. No doubt I had experienced this?

I said I had, and described a few of my awful moments. Dr. Walsh nodded. His expression was sympathetic—he had the perfect bedside manner that seems to have vanished from medicine in the age of the specialist. The other consequence, he continued, was that the thickened muscle of the bladder wall would be working too hard once the prostate was removed and the urethra freed from obstruction. The bladder would not get the message that things had changed. It would still be pushing hard, but this time against a single, damaged sphincter instead of two undamaged ones, and at first, inevitably, the remaining sphincter's ability to hold back the flow of urine would be overwhelmed. Dr. Walsh quickly sketched the bladder, like an upside-down jar, and showed how the walls became thickened due to muscle buildup. I could not help thinking that he must be a superb teacher—he had a natural gift for explaining things in the simplest terms. In a few words he had made clear to me something that nobody had ever bothered to explain before.

Dr. Walsh's pager buzzed, summoning him away from us briefly.

"What do you think of him?" I asked Margaret.

She had on her dark glasses—a sure sign that she was hiding her feelings. "You have to make up your own mind," she said. "I'm sure he's a good surgeon, but it's up to you."

"I don't think he's going to take me," I said.

"What makes you think that?"

"The way he said that Memorial was a fine hospital. And now this business about how he doesn't like to operate on a prostate as enlarged as mine. . . . He's going to say no. I feel it in my bones."

I *did* feel it in my bones—and my guts—too. It was strange. Up to the point where I actually met Dr. Walsh, I had been perfectly content to have Russo perform the operation. Now that I was at Johns Hopkins, I had the feeling that my life depended on Dr. Walsh's decision.

He returned, apologized, and resumed his place. Summoning up my nerve, I asked him if the enlargement of my prostate would preclude his taking my case. Dr. Walsh shook his head, perhaps in surprise. Not at all, he said, he would be delighted to operate on me. I was so relieved that I didn't even realize until later that I had already made *my* decision, just as Margaret had guessed I would.

I asked Dr. Walsh about incontinence, particularly in view of my enlarged prostate. He did not think I should be concerned. Even with a large prostate like mine, the odds were good that continence would return. In any event, he pointed out, given what I had told him about my urinary problems over the past few years, my quality of life in that respect was already compromised. Sooner or later, I would have needed surgery to open up the urethra, even without the cancer.

And sex? I asked. He could see no reason why I should not be able to enjoy sex fully after the surgery, and he would do everything he could to make that possible. Some things would change, of course. But had I not already experienced changes, frankly? At sixty, my sexual function was nothing like it had been when I was seventeen, or even thirty. No man's is. Our sex life would be different, there was no denying that, but "different" did not have to mean less rich or fulfilling—indeed, one of his primary objectives was to make sure of that.

These were exactly the words I wanted to hear. Dr. Russo had been more cautious, emphasizing the importance of getting rid of the cancer as opposed to preserving sexual function, while the radiologist had been downright pessimistic.

I told Dr. Walsh that I had been looking at the numbers, particularly the ten-year survival rate, and I pulled from my briefcase a few of the papers the radiologist had given me. Dr. Walsh's geniality vanished instantly. He grabbed the papers out of my hands and flipped through them. "Who gave you these?" he asked.

I explained that the radiologist I had consulted at Memorial had offered them—though I was cautious enough not to say that he had been trying to show me that his numbers were as good as Dr. Walsh's, or better. Dr. Walsh stabbed at the markings in yellow fluorescent Hi-Liter. Who had marked the papers up?, he wanted to know.

Some of them, of course, had been heavily gone over by the radiologist in his initial burst of enthusiasm, but others had been highlighted, more neatly, by me as I tried to make sense of them. Still, it seemed expedient to let the radiologist take the full responsibility, since *he* wasn't going to be operated on by Dr. Walsh.

Dr. Walsh returned the papers. I should put them away and forget about them, he said. Better yet, I should throw them away. Numbers meant nothing. Each case was different. I was an individual, not a statistic.

That, too, was exactly what I wanted to hear: that I was an individual, not a statistic. All the same, I felt a slight ripple of guilt. Everyone (except his former patients) had told me that I *must* ask Dr. Walsh about his numbers, and compare them to those of Dr. Russo and the radiologist, and to the average. *Whoever* the surgeon was, I had a right, an obligation even, to know what his rate of success was, how long his patients lived, how many of them needed further treatment, even, more embarrassingly, if any of them died in surgery.

This had struck me as difficult to do—rather like comparative shopping for a surgeon with a copy of the medical equivalent of *Consumer's Digest* in hand—but in the light of Dr. Walsh's self-confidence and take-charge attitude, his numbers, whatever they were, seemed simply irrelevant.

—⁓—

I WAS LUCKY to have Dr. Walsh as my surgeon, but I think most men in my position should do a more thorough job of research before deciding anything as important as this. Important decisions should not be made on instinct or in a hurry, least of all in a vacuum. After all, a radical prostatectomy is the reverse of emergency surgery. There is plenty of time to consult with surgeons, to ask for their numbers and study them, and to make an evaluation based on something more than a firm handshake. Of course, for a lot of people—the vast majority—the choice of a surgeon is limited for all sorts of reasons. Health-care plans, increasingly, tend to determine the choice, particularly in HMOs, and men living in small towns, away from the big urban medical centers, are likely to be faced with a narrow choice among local urologists. Not everyone can afford to travel to Baltimore to consult with Patrick Walsh, or to Houston to see Peter Scardino—besides which, the local man (or woman, though women are rare in urology) may be perfectly good.

As it turns out, a great many men simply accept what their urologist tells them without questioning him at all, except, perhaps, to ask if their health insurance will cover the full cost of the procedure. This is a mistake. At a very minimum, a patient ought to ask his prospective surgeon whether or not he performs the "nerve-sparing" procedure, how many he has done, and what percentage of his patients have recovered potency, as well as what his ten-year survival rate is. Surely it makes sense to spend at least as much time reading up on a procedure that will change the rest of your life—and determine how long it will be, as well—as you would before buying a new car. The more you know, and the more questions you ask, the more likely you will be to have a successful surgical experience and recuperation. You can't expect a busy surgeon to educate you about prostate cancer in only one session, let alone to tell you what questions you ought to be asking him.

—⁓—

THOUGH I FAILED to question Dr. Walsh about his ten-year survival numbers, I more than made up for it with questions that concerned me far more, perhaps because they seemed more immediate. How long, for instance, would I be in the hospital?

I should count on five days, Dr. Walsh said.

That seemed to me a lot shorter than the average, I said. Yes, Dr. Walsh agreed, but the key thing was that he performed the procedure in about two hours. I recalled that Dr. Russo had told me the operation would take about four hours. How had Dr. Walsh managed to halve it? One of the answers, it turned out, was that Dr. Walsh performed his operation with an epidural rather than a full general anesthetic. I would not feel a thing, he promised. The epidural was safer, made the recovery time much shorter, and made the procedure less traumatic. The other answer, though Dr. Walsh did not say so directly, lay in his special expertise and skill. This was *his* operation, after all, he had performed nearly 1,600 of them, and he had it down to a fine art.

Did he pause to have a biopsy done on the lymph nodes? I wanted to know. Absolutely. Tissue from the lymph nodes was removed and dissected before the removal of the prostate. If the cancer had spread to them, then he would generally not go on with the operation, but he saw no reason to believe that would be my case.

I wanted to know more about epidural versus full general anesthetic—somehow the idea of being *conscious,* however dimly, during major surgery did not appeal to me, though I was aware that general anesthesia is usually the most dangerous part of any surgery. I understood there was every reason to prefer an epidural—it would be safer, and far less traumatic to the body—except that I had a kind of holy fear of the very idea. The whole notion of a spinal tap had always filled me with horror, and a spinal anesthetic (which is what an epidural basically is) could not be so very different. We all have our areas of irrational fear: with some people it's the dark, or heights, or dentistry; with me it had always been the notion of an injection into my spinal column, perhaps because it was something I had heard about as a child—and here was Pat Walsh, calmly proposing a spinal to me as if it were something I should be pleased about!

I wondered if there was any way out of the spinal anesthetic, but it appeared it was not optional—besides which, the epidural catheter, inserted into my spinal column for the anesthetic, would also be used, it turned out, for giving me painkillers after the surgery. I would be linked up to an IV drip and be provided with a "pain button," enabling me to control the frequency of my "pain shots." Patients suffered less pain when they felt they were in control of the situation, rather than having to wait for a nurse to give them an injection or call for her when the pain proved bothersome.

I liked the sound of that—one of the few dim memories I retained of my appendectomy was pushing the button again and again for the nurse when I was in pain, with no result. On the other hand, I wondered how I would deal with pain once I was home.

I would have none, Dr. Walsh said. In fact, I would be free of pain long before I even left the hospital. Really, I should not worry about pain at all, in fact, since almost none was involved.

I liked the sound of that even more, though I took it with a grain of salt. One of Dr. Walsh's patients, as a matter of fact, had told me that in *his* case the first couple of days were terrible, reaching a climax on the third night after the operation, after which he began to feel better fast. That sounded plausible, but I decided not to bring it up with Dr. Walsh. How, I wondered instead, would I get home after the operation? Margaret and I had been concerned about that.

Dr. Walsh brushed away our concern. I would be fine. His patients left the hospital and went home every day, some of them to California, Europe, or even the Middle East. I should not travel by car, certainly, because of the bumping and jarring, but I would be perfectly able to go home by plane or train.

And aftercare at home? Would I need a nurse? Dr. Walsh didn't think so. Nothing much was involved except emptying the catheter bag at regular intervals. A Foley catheter would be inserted during surgery, and I would retain it for about three weeks after the operation. My local urologist could remove it when the time came. Dr. Walsh saw no reason why I couldn't empty my own catheter bag; patients were taught how to look after their catheter by the nursing staff before being sent home.

This sounded optimistic to me. I made a mental note to explore the availability of home health care in Dutchess County, New York. The catheter gave me pause. I couldn't imagine what it would be like to have one for three weeks, or what it would feel like when it was removed. One patient I'd spoken with had mentioned that it was the worst feeling he'd ever experienced; others merely remarked that it was a deeply unpleasant sensation.

I tried to think of further questions, but my mind had gone blank. So far I had put off thinking about surgery, on the grounds that until I had my second opinion from Dr. Walsh I couldn't decide anything. Now the inevitability of it was coming home to me. There was not going to be any last-minute reprieve. The next time I saw Dr. Walsh he would be wearing surgical scrubs and a mask and I would be stretched out on his operating table, with—I shuddered at the image—an epidural in my back. It was clear that we had already used up as much of Dr. Walsh's time as we were entitled to. We all rose to say good-bye. We should stop by and speak to his secretary on the way out, Dr. Walsh said, taking my decision for granted. She would give me a date for the surgery—he suspected that it would have to be after Thanksgiving, in about four weeks, given his schedule and the need for me to give three pints of my own blood in case they were needed during the operation—again, I could not give more than one pint a week. His secretary would also give me instructions for what to do between now and the morning of surgery, and I should read these carefully—we *both* should, in fact, he added, giving Margaret a meaningful glance.

I looked at Margaret, too, since I knew she had all sorts of questions, but she appeared to have been struck dumb. Perhaps she, too, was feeling the inevitability of the thing. She had accompanied me to three consultations, looking for answers—now we had the answers, except for the answer to the big question: *Would it work?*

Dr. Walsh and I shook hands—he had a strong, firm grip. To my surprise, he put his hand on my shoulder and looked me right in the eye. "Don't worry," he said. "I'm going to take care of you." He seemed perfectly confident, his pale blue eyes absolutely sincere. "I'm going to give you the best operation I can," he added. "You'll be fine, I promise."

Then he was gone, hurrying out the door in his starched white coat.

When we left Johns Hopkins for the airport, after filling out innumerable forms, I had a date: November 29, right after Thanksgiving, exactly four weeks away.

I felt a curious sense of relief. The decision had been made at last—had simply fallen into place, without any real debate on my part. I had put my fate in Dr. Walsh's hands, and he seemed to have no doubts at all about his ability to deal with it. All I had to do was give a pint of blood a week for the next three weeks, and have no second thoughts.

PART TWO

SURGERY

11

BUT OF COURSE IT WAS HARD TO THINK ABOUT ANYTHING ELSE. LUCK-ily for me, the effort of preparing for the known—an absence from the office of at least six to eight weeks—was enough to keep my mind off the *un*known for long periods of the day. There were also plenty of things to do on the personal front before I underwent surgery.

The first was to meet with somebody from my firm's Human Resources department, to make sure that I was covered by my company health insurance and, perhaps more important, that the insurer was kept informed and accepted my choice of Dr. Walsh. Over the years, I had made scant use of our medical coverage, but it was now going to be put to the test. I am happy to report that it performed flawlessly (and promptly), but it taught me one lesson: hitherto, I had not paid much attention to my health insurance; henceforth, I would take good care to understand exactly how it worked, rather than having to undergo a crash course.

I also decided to draw up a living will, giving Margaret the right to tell the doctor not to prolong my life under certain circumstances.

This was more difficult, since she didn't even want to *hear* about it, but I had read enough horror stories to insist. Once again, it isn't something that can be left to the very last moment, unless you're planning to turn up for your surgery with your lawyer. A living will, if it's to be of any use, has to be part of your preoperative file. I studied a few examples and chose one of the simpler ones, which made it clear that I did not wish to be kept alive by extraordinary or artificial means, or revived if it was certain that I was dying. I sent a signed copy to Dr. Walsh's office and gave the original to Margaret to keep handy.

It was a small, solemn moment between us, as we briefly faced the possibility that I might die. Margaret and I are not untypical—neither of us wanted to think about death, and we had never really discussed it. Now there was no avoiding it. Admittedly, the likelihood of death or a coma during a surgical procedure is remote, but these things can (and do) happen. The living will made me feel better about the surgery, though I recognized that it placed upon Margaret an awful responsibility.

It was the first of many such burdens, small and large, for despite the story about Dr. Walsh's cartoonist patient who had been back to work in his hospital bed only a few days after surgery, I had a premonition that in the aftermath of surgery I wasn't going to be interested in anything much outside my own body for a while. I made sure Margaret had a copy of my will and a detailed, up-to-date list of assets; I had a power of attorney drawn up in her name; I put everything that she might need to know down on paper—and asked myself, as I was doing so, why I had waited for a medical crisis to do it. Another lesson for the future, I decided—if there was one.

Dealing with work was another problem. I may as well confess that I am a compulsive workaholic, and always have been. The idea of *letting go,* of delegating, of being out of touch for several weeks, seemed to me unimaginable, and yet it had to be faced realistically. Everybody I'd spoken with who had undergone a radical prostatectomy agreed upon one thing, if nothing else: it would take all my energy and attention to recover from the operation—even if I *wanted* to think about work, I wouldn't be able to. The first sign of recovery, in fact, would be when I began to take an interest again in what was going on at the office.

Of course, I didn't believe a word of it. I was made, I told myself, of sterner stuff than that! I made plans to have my laptop brought down to Johns Hopkins, so I could be in touch with the office by E-mail and paperless faxing; I made a list of manuscripts I would have sent down to me, so I could read and edit in bed. Just to be on the safe side, I delegated a lot of my projects to other editors, but I thought of this as a backup. As things turned out, it was fortunate that I did this.

And what can have been on my mind, I wonder now, when I decided to take all three volumes of Douglas Southall Freeman's *Lee's Lieutenants* down to Baltimore, or Simon Schama's weighty *Citizens*?

—⁂—

ON THE OTHER hand, some things I did would turn out to be indispensable. A call to one of my local hospitals, St. Francis, in Poughkeepsie, put me in touch with St. Francis's Homecare Service and opened up a new world to me. Never having been seriously sick, I had no idea of the range of services available to a patient recovering from surgery. The general denunciation of the American health-care system that accompanied the failed attempt to produce a national health system had led me to believe that our country's way of doing things didn't work; that the Canadian system, whatever it might be, was better; that faced with a real medical crisis you were virtually on your own. It was soon apparent that this was not the case. A kindly and efficient woman at St. Francis quickly filled me in on what she could do for me—as well as giving me, at last, a reasonably accurate view of what I would need when I got home. She did not share Dr. Walsh's belief that I would need no help. She would provide an RN who would visit me once a day, to begin with. The nurse would monitor my vital signs and my condition, and report back on a regular basis to my doctor.

The woman at St. Francis also put me in touch with a home nursing service, which would provide a nurse's aide several hours every day. She felt I would need both a visiting nurse and a nurse's aide, at least at first. She then got in touch with Dr. Walsh and with my insurance company, to make sure everything was in place and waiting on my return.

She said that I should fix up one bathroom with a hand shower, since I would be unable to bathe until the incision healed, as well as with handrails and a nonslip bathtub seat. I would need big surgical pads, surgical tape (lots of both), surgical alcohol, Betadyne soap, Q-Tips, antibiotic ointment, a rubber-backed waterproof pad to put on the bed (and several more to put on chairs, just in case), plenty of disposable pads, and a couple of packages of disposable adult incontinence pants (I resisted the idea of thinking of them as "diapers," but that's the part of the supermarket where they're found). Washable, nonslip, foam-backed carpets or pads should be placed in strategic areas, both to prevent my slipping and to deal with any "accidents." I wrote it all down obediently—recovery was beginning to take on a clearer picture, though not one I liked much.

Still, what impressed me most was how helpful she—and everybody else at my local level—was. Did I need the nurse's aide to do my shopping for me, or cooking, or laundry? I needed none of these things, in fact, but the very idea that they were available, and at a fairly modest cost, most if not all of which would be reimbursed under my company's health-insurance plan, surprised me. Far from being a wilderness where social services to the ill were concerned, Dutchess County, which is by no means atypical, turned out to have layer after layer of services, so much so that it would eventually seem to me that the job of one half the county's population was looking after the other half.

Where did we ever get the idea that this wasn't so, I wondered, that health care was better in England or Canada? (I can't speak for Canada, but I have lived in England, and if I were sick there, the first thing I'd do would be to get on a plane to New York.) I think the blame lies partly with the media, which prints only the *bad* news and ignores the extraordinary vitality and range of health-care services available throughout most of the United States, and partly with people like me, who have simply never bothered to pursue the system and find out just what they're entitled to. In the next few months I was to experience everything from emergency-room treatment to our local volunteer fire company's emergency ambulance service, and the level of commitment, cheerfulness, and efficiency of the people I came into contact with never failed to impress and amaze me.

Two things, however, must be said. The first is that you cannot leave this kind of thing until the last moment; the second is that you have to ask, to make the calls, to track down the services that are available where you live.

I am a great believer in this kind of preparation. In part, it's a way of admitting to oneself that it's *going* to happen, for better or for worse—the boxes of surgical pads and the packages of adult diapers in the closet bring home the reality of the thing; in part, I find that careful preparation—thinking ahead—calms one's fears. The question is no longer "What's going to happen to me?"—which may not be answerable—but "Am I ready for it?"—which is easier to deal with. Practical, day-to-day, logistical problems are a lot easier to solve than big philosophical ones.

It's also something that one's entire family can join in—a project which brings home to everyone, even children, what's involved, and yet makes it clear that it isn't *permanent*, that recuperation is a stage to go through, with full recovery at the end of it. A lot of people might feel shame—or at least embarrassment—at shopping for adult incontinence pants, but I think this is a mistake. If you're going to have to wear them, you may as well admit to it, at any rate to your nearest and dearest, if not necessarily to your colleagues. Incontinence, while no fun, is a lot less scary than dying of cancer.

—⁓—

I FOUND GIVING the blood strangely soothing, much as I dislike needles. My local blood bank in New York City turned out to be a surprisingly cheerful place, particularly once they knew I was giving my own blood for a cancer operation. While the decor was unmistakably big-city urban-medical, the atmosphere was partylike, and the procedure, for once as promised, totally painless. I *enjoyed* lying there, cradled in sympathy, while a pint of my blood was pumped into a transparent plastic bag, to be frozen and forwarded to Johns Hopkins. I met interesting people—one, a New York–based movie producer with whom I exchanged cards and PSA levels, was also going to be operated on by Dr. Walsh—and afterward I was helped into a cheery canteen, where they served cranberry juice, granola bars, and candy, and made sure that I didn't leave if I was feeling faint.

Where, I wondered (as I had at Memorial Sloan-Kettering), are these sullen, unhappy, bureaucracy-strangled health-care professionals that we read about, who treat every patient as if he or she were just a number? These people genuinely *cared* about me—they were in my corner, and did nothing to hide it.

There is a certain clubbiness to illness that is one of its few saving graces. At the blood bank, all the autologous donors (those giving blood for their own eventual use) have a known problem and a scheduled date for some kind of major procedure. You can talk about your own troubles and listen to other people's, which is no small comfort, since at this stage of things, a couple of weeks or so before surgery, I had pretty well exhausted the number of friends and acquaintances who wanted to hear about my cancer.

At the New York blood bank, donors are given a small, red plastic lapel pin in the shape of a drop of blood, and I was soon sporting mine proudly. I still have four of them, one for each session, and the memories of those long, dreamy afternoons, away from the intrusions of phone calls—playing hooky, as it were, but with a purpose— are surprisingly pleasant ones. The weather was good—Indian summer—and I invariably strolled home, window-shopping on the way, stopping on Sixty-eighth Street, just off Madison Avenue, for a cappuccino, and at the Madison Avenue Book Shop, a block or so farther up, to chat with Arthur Loeb and look at the new stock. I, who never waste time in New York City, found myself turning, once a week, into a flaneur, a boulevardier, and rather enjoyed the feeling—though it was an illusion, of course. Far from being a carefree stroller, I had cancer. I couldn't help wondering if this would be the last time in my life I'd enjoy an aimless late afternoon in New York—and perhaps, looking back, it was exactly that thought that made me enjoy it so much.

I think there is a lot to be said for having the best time you can before surgery. There is nothing like pleasure for taking one's mind off things like cancer surgery; more important, it's worth keeping in mind that whatever your surgeon may say, it will be a long time—if ever—before you can do any of those things you enjoy.

Sex, for example, will undoubtedly be different after surgery, even assuming that potency returns, which, in a sizable number of cases, it may not. There *is* sex after radical prostatectomy, absolutely, for most men, but at the very least it is going to be more difficult to get an erection (and may require special aids, devices, or medication, about which more later), and orgasm will be dry—that is, without ejaculation or any fluid emission. Not the end of the world, as urologists never tire of pointing out, and a lot better than dying of prostate cancer, but still, not quite the same as the sex one used to have.

It makes sense to have fun in the face of what is surely not going to be any fun at all, which is not to suggest that you should indulge in an orgy (even assuming your partner is in a mood to do so) but *is* to suggest that you should try to make these weeks of waiting as agreeable as possible *for both of you*. It is better (and healthier) to stack up a few happy memories for the bad days ahead than to spend the weeks before the operation brooding about one's fate.

—⁓—

I DID MY best not to think about what was coming, sometimes successfully, sometimes not. I *did* take the time to write a long letter to Dr. Russo explaining that I had decided to have my surgery performed by Dr. Walsh; that he mustn't feel this in any way indicated a lack of respect on my part for him or for Memorial Hospital; and that I would always be grateful for the time and care he and his colleagues had given to my case. In the end, I hadn't made my choice *rationally,* by carefully comparing the numbers, but *intuitively,* based on Dr. Walsh's extraordinary (though well-contained) self-confidence. It may be that this is as good a way as any to decide these things, but I am a great believer in not worrying about things that are already decided upon. After a certain point, *"Che sera, sera"* is my motto.

A part of me was behaving rationally—getting my desk in order, making sure that Margaret had enough money to pay bills, storing my car away (Dr. Walsh discouraged patients from driving until eight weeks after the operation), discreetly picking up little necessities for a hospital stay (slippers, a robe, an electric razor)—while the rest of me tried to take what amounted to a mini-vacation. Margaret and I took long walks, caught up on a lot of movies, ate out a lot. We did not talk about the coming operation much—not so much consciously avoiding the subject as accepting that everything that could be discussed *had* been discussed.

I can't remember any other time of my life, except for the period of recuperation itself, when I ever felt more detached from what I would normally regard as urgent or pressing concerns. Neither office crises nor world affairs seemed very important when compared to what was going to happen to me on November twenty-ninth, or to what was presumably taking place in my prostate at that very moment. I felt the kind of diminished interest in everyday matters that must, I suppose, affect people taking up a monastic life, or deciding to give up everything and sail single-handed around the world. It was not an uncomfortable feeling—a loosening of ties in preparation for an adventure or, at the very least, a change.

Xanax had been prescribed for me, just in case I might feel anxiety, but the truth was that I didn't, although I did suffer from occasional nightmares, most of them having to do with surgery.

They were either dreams in which I watched while a surgeon, faceless behind his mask and glasses, cut me open without anesthesia, or in which I felt myself dying—actually *watching* my own death, as it were, from outside my own body, while at the same time undergoing it. I did not experience warm white light, a sensation of well-being, or friendly voices coming to greet me as I passed over—on the contrary, I experienced death as a grim and scary business, not so much painful as lonely.

Happily, one Xanax at bedtime took care of these nightmares, and I slept like a baby. Every morning I woke up feeling fine, ran a couple of miles, ate a healthy breakfast, congratulated myself on feeling 100 percent fit, and had to persuade myself, against all the evidence, that I was in fact sicker than I had ever been, or *expected* to be. It wasn't so much that it didn't seem *fair*—nothing is, after all—it didn't even seem *possible*.

PERPAPS THE HARDEST thing was finally going public with the news that I had cancer. Of course, a lot of people already knew, since I had made no big secret of it—strongly against some people's advice—but now that I had a date for surgery, I felt it was important to announce the fact myself, rather than having it spread through book publishing in the form of rumors.

It's a tricky thing, this business of whom you tell, and when. I had told my son, Chris, as soon as I received the bad news about the biopsies, whereas I had shillied and shallied and finally decided *not* to tell my mother. She is an active eighty-two-year-old, but still, eighty-two is eighty-two: I thought it would be kinder to tell her about it after it was over, rather than have her worrying about the surgery. I had told the people closest to me at work at the very beginning, as I've said. Now I decided that I should break the news to all my colleagues at our weekly meeting.

I do not normally suffer from stage fright, perhaps because my mother was an actress; actually, I usually enjoy public speaking. This time, however, my hands were trembling and my throat was dry. I wanted to strike the right balance between optimism and realism, not an easy thing to do in front of twenty or thirty people assembled around a big table in the Simon & Schuster conference room.

Toward the end of the meeting, Carolyn Reidy, the president of Simon & Schuster's trade division, read the next Sunday's *New York Times* bestseller list aloud—something of a ritual—then said that I had a private announcement to make. I could see from the expression on people's faces that a lot of them thought, either with dismay or pleasure, that I was about to announce my resignation. Oddly enough, it felt that way to me, too, perhaps because that is usually what such announcements are about—I had heard countless such speeches myself, with varying degrees of emotion, delivered in this same room, across this same table.

"It's not what you're thinking," I began. I paused for a moment, then decided to plunge right in, the quicker the better. "I have cancer." I let it sink in. The word seemed to resonate in the air. Now that I'd spoken it, I felt better. "Some of you, a few, already know that, but I want you *all* to know, first of all because I think of you as friends, and also because I'm going to be out of the office for at least eight weeks, so some of you are going to have to take up the slack and help out on my books while I'm away. I know how busy you all are, and how little you need an additional burden, so I thank you in advance. As for my cancer, it's prostate cancer. It's not the worst kind you can have, and the good news is that it doesn't appear to have spread. I'm sure a lot of you have a relative, perhaps even a father, who's had prostate cancer, so I don't need to tell you that while it's no fun, there's a very good chance of surviving it just fine if it's caught early on, which mine was."

It was hard to read what they were thinking. Hardly anybody seemed to want to make eye contact with me, but then, if I'd been sitting where they were, I don't suppose I would have been seeking out eye contact either. "I've decided to be operated on at Johns Hopkins, in Baltimore, by Patrick Walsh, who's one of the great surgeons in America, so I'm in good hands. My surgery is on November twenty-ninth, right after Thanksgiving. This isn't a secret, by the way. I just didn't want to announce it like this until I knew what the date of the operation was. Please feel free to tell the people who work for you, or people on the outside. I'd just as soon that everybody heard the truth, which is what this is, instead of a bunch of rumors."

Was I doing the right thing? Some of my friends wanted the company to put out a press release. I refused. I am not, after all, the president of the United States. I don't owe it to anybody to put out a health bulletin; besides which, it seems to me a pretentious thing to do. Others were still urging me to keep my cancer as secret as I could, for the sake of my career. This is not, alas, such an absurd concern as it may sound. It is not unheard of for a company to fire somebody the moment it discovers he (or she) has cancer—allegedly, of course, for other reasons—which means that if you've been diagnosed with cancer and admit to the fact, you may lose not only your job but also your health coverage. I did not think this would happen to me, and I was right—no company could have been more supportive than Simon & Schuster—but it *does* happen, as I was later to discover. Cancer brings with it many fears, and not all of them are about death or dying.

I had one more thing to add: "I just want to say to every man in this room that if you don't know what your PSA is, *find out!* Today! You have to know. You have to make sure your physician examines your prostate and takes your PSA at least once a year. It's a matter of life and death. Yours."

I thanked everybody for listening so patiently, gathered up my papers, and left the room. I felt absolutely exhausted. It was the hardest speech I'd ever made, but I was glad I'd done it. It was so much easier when it was all out in the open and everyone knew. Also, it astonished me to discover just how many people *did*, in fact, have relatives with prostate cancer. For the next few days my office was like a consulting room, as man after man knocked on my door and came in to ask me about prostate cancer, or tell me what his PSA level was, while woman after woman came in to share with me the story of what happened to her father when he found out he had prostate cancer. It was as if prostate cancer was some kind of rite of passage for the over-fifty-year-old man, so widespread did it appear to be. I felt a certain strangeness. I thought of myself as youthful, if not young, but I was clearly classified in the same age group as the fathers of most of the women in my office, or, in only a few cases, thank God, their *grand*fathers! Unfortunately, I couldn't very well ask them if their fathers had regained their sexual potency or whether they were still incontinent.

—⚭—

THE DAY THE office closed for the Thanksgiving vacation, Margaret came to pick me up. I made my good-byes. I had tried to keep a stiff upper lip for several weeks, but this time I couldn't do it. So many people wished me good luck, embraced me, assured me that they would be thinking of me, or praying for me, that I could feel tears in my eyes by the time we reached the elevator. I was sure—well, almost sure, anyway—that I would be coming back here, but when, and in what shape? I felt as if I were closing a chapter of my life, and of course the truth is, I was. Before and after prostate-cancer surgery, as I would discover, are different worlds, and you cannot imagine the second when you are still in the first.

Thanksgiving weekend Margaret and I spent together quietly, trying not to think about what lay in store for both of us. I had no doubt that Margaret's role would be as difficult as mine—perhaps in some ways *more* difficult, because everyone's attention is naturally focused on the patient's problems, whereas the fears, problems, and feelings of the patient's spouse or companion go largely ignored. It's not just that sickness often results in a reversal of roles—the strong person in a relationship may suddenly become the weak one, the caretaker needs caring for, the person who has always looked after things now needs looking after, and so forth—it also creates feelings that can't be acknowledged, that can't, perhaps, even be admitted to oneself.

It's hard to argue with a man who has cancer, and even harder to be angry with him, and yet women often do feel anger, inevitably—

anger that their lives are being upset, anger at being abandoned, however innocently; for serious illness is a kind of abandonment, in which the patient becomes totally immersed in his own case, in his own health, his own needs.

"How could he *do* this to me?" is what a lot of women must feel, yet they cannot say it out loud, or even *think* it, without feeling guilty. Fear—fear of the unknown, fear that he's going to die, fear that even if he *doesn't* die he will emerge from all this a different person—breeds anger, as fear always does, made stronger in this case by the fact that it can't be expressed.

It's strange, I think, that nobody has written about this side of prostate cancer. Surgeons—mostly men, since urology remains a largely male specialty—ignore it completely. In their view, the woman's role is to be supportive during the surgery and caring afterward, part cheerleader, part Red Cross nurse. To judge by the books on prostate cancer and the advice to patients handed out prior to surgery, one would suppose that every marriage is a bedrock-solid equal partnership, but in real life this is hardly always the case.

The truth is that prostate cancer inevitably involves the most difficult and frequently unresolved areas of a relationship. The direct threat to a man's sexual identity and ability to perform can hardly fail to have an effect on the relationship. Women must ask themselves how impotence, if it results, will affect the relationship, how they will feel about it themselves, how it will change things. Questions are likely to include: "What will he be like if he can't have sex?"; "How will I feel about that?"; "How will we handle it?"

It goes without saying that men who can talk to their wives freely about their innermost feelings and fears, not to mention their sexuality, will do better in facing the problems of prostate cancer than those for whom this is not the case, but, frankly, how many people can say that about their marriage? Mostly, these are exactly the subjects that men find it difficult to talk about and share with their wives. The mere fact of being diagnosed as having prostate cancer is not likely to transform the average husband into a sensitive, articulate man, eager to discuss his darkest fears at length with his wife.

You can get all the information you need—though it takes some doing—about Gleason scores, the different ways of attacking the disease, and so forth, but when it comes to what it's going to do to your marriage, you're on your own, and I don't have any doubt that this adds considerably to the level of anxiety on both sides.

An example: about fifteen years ago, I underwent a vasectomy. Margaret and I didn't want children (I have a son by a former marriage), and both of us were concerned about the risks for her of staying on the Pill. The operation, billed as a simple, painless, in-office procedure, turned out to be long, bloody, and very painful—an exception, I have no doubt, to the rule, but still a memorably unpleasant experience.

Lo and behold, no sooner did I start reading up on prostate cancer than I discovered that men who have had a vasectomy may have a higher incidence of prostate cancer than those who have not. To be exact, a 1990 report on three thousand patients with prostate cancer found that "the rate of prostate cancer, present in 610 men, was *twice* as high for men who had undergone vasectomies."[*] This is about the same percentage as was found in a Johns Hopkins study of men whose fathers or brothers had prostate cancer.[†]

Researchers established "an association," not a "risk factor," which, in layman's terms, merely means that the case, while compelling and worthy of further research, remains unproven.[‡] Still, I couldn't help

[*] Study reported in the *American Journal of Epidemiology* by Dr. Curtis Mettlin, Roswell Park Cancer Institute, Buffalo, New York, as quoted in *The Well-Informed Patient's Guide to Prostate Problems,* by Charles E. Shapiro, M.D., and Kathleen Doheny, Dell, 1993.
[†] Gary D. Steinberg, M.D., James Buchanan Brady Urological Institute, Johns Hopkins, as published in *The Prostate.*
[‡] While the vasectomy thesis remains conjectural, proof *is* rapidly accumulating that genetics plays a significant role in prostate cancer. Memorial Sloan-Kettering's Department of Human Genetics already lists prostate cancer high among those that are genetically driven, and the department's Clinical Genetics Service, under the guidance of Service Chief Kenneth Offit, M.D., P.M.H., is in the forefront of tracing a medical "family tree," which can be used to determine whether family members are truly at risk of getting cancer (including prostate cancer), thus opening up the possibility of cancer prevention for those determined to be at risk.

wondering, given the numbers in the 1990 study, whether my vasectomy might not have been the cause of my cancer, though the answer appears to be almost certainly not.

Such questions as these are normal; prostate cancer by definition touches what is likely to be the most sensitive part of any marriage—the sexual relationship—and in the weeks before the surgery, if you are taking the surgical route, there are going to be a lot of strong emotions going on under the surface. Some men may feel a regret for opportunities they turned down; while both women and men alike may wonder what will become of the marriage if the man loses his potency. Blame, fear, mixed emotions, regrets—it is important to recognize that all these are *legitimate* feelings in the face of something that is certainly going to change your life, either temporarily or permanently. There is a value to smiling through it bravely—the famous stiff upper lip—but that should not preclude a couple's ability to face all this emotional distress squarely. At the very least, there ought to be some discussion of the issue of impotence, which is the thing that most men are afraid of (death tends to run a close second). *Not* talking about the possibility is a mistake.

In my case, I made sure that Margaret read all the material about impotence in the books I had found, however reluctant she was to do so. We naturally hoped this would *not* be the outcome, but at least we knew and understood what could be done about it if it did happen, as well as what would be acceptable to both of us in the way of sexual aids (about which, more later). Once you've talked about it frankly with your partner, you can put the possibility of impotence in the back of your mind, rather than letting it become an obsession.

You cannot leave this to your doctor, or expect that a busy surgeon is going to have the time to transform himself into a marriage counselor or sex therapist—besides which, the recommendations of a man, in *this* area, may not make any sense at all to a woman. The mere fact that urologists operate below the belt, in the region of desire, does not necessarily convey any special understanding of sexuality, or sympathy toward women—indeed, some urologists have a tendency to think of the sexual organs in terms of "plumbing," and many of their solutions for sexual difficulties involve more surgery and the implantation of prosthetic devices, ignoring the fact that couples can very often find their own ways of dealing with these problems. In any case, a woman's view of what is desirable in this area may be very different from a man's, let alone a male surgeon's.

The period *before* surgery will determine more than anything else (except perhaps the surgeon's skill) the speed with which the patient will recover and how he will feel about it. *Expect* quarrels and disagreements, by the way—volatile issues are at stake. Ignore the Goody Two-Shoes approach that presumes a little good sex and hand-holding are all it takes to prepare for what's to come. What's needed is a strong, united front—and a realistic, clear-eyed approach to the problems that may follow surgery.

Be assured, prostate cancer will try your soul and the soul of the partner who loves you, and subject your marriage to the acid test of facing some of life's more difficult problems. Faced courageously—and people have more courage, generally speaking, than they give themselves credit for—it can strengthen a marriage and, surprisingly, show you that not only is there life after prostate cancer, but that the best may still be to come.

━━━

AT HOME, I could hardly fail to notice the preparations for my return after surgery. Everywhere I looked there was evidence of careful, thoughtful preparation, for which I am still grateful. Our friends Roxanne and Richard Bacon had been busy. Since ours is an old (1784) house, without showers, Richard had rigged up a bathtub with a shower curtain, a hand shower, and a shower seat, and he fixed handles to the wall so I could steady myself; there was also a no-slip mat on the floor. In the bedroom was a modem for my laptop, so that I could be in contact with the office while I rested, and there was another next to the sofa in my study, so that I could lie down and rest while I was working.

Armed with the list I had drawn up during my conversation about nursing, I made an exploratory trip to my local pharmacy, John's Apothecary, which makes something of a specialty of older patients, and stood in awe at the vast range of products for the incontinent. Obviously, I was about to join one of the largest minorities in the country, perhaps a little before my time. I consoled myself with the thought that everybody who lives long enough is going to end up shopping for disposable adult diapers, urinals, and leakproof mattress covers.

John led me through the whole range of products with tact and a salesman's enthusiasm. There was your basic Depends adult diaper, a bit on the bulky side, but "100 percent leakproof," even for full incontinence. I would need these after I got home, in case my catheter leaked, as most did, and for an indeterminate time after the catheter was removed. Then, he went on, holding them up, you had your Attends briefs, absorbent, less bulky, held on by two reusable elastic straps, and looking like a heavily padded bikini bottom. I would graduate to these when I had regained some continence. Of course, if I coughed, stood up suddenly, sneezed, or laughed hard, I would have an involuntary "spurt" of urine, but the Attends would cope with this, if I got his meaning. I nodded, assuring him that I did. After that, I would move on to your Sir Dignity brief, looking like a pair of Jockey shorts, but with a plastic pouch in front into which an absorbent pad was fitted. At first I would be changing pads a lot, but pretty soon most men found that all they needed to do was to carry a spare pad around in the breast pocket of their jacket, just in case of accidents. He held a pair up, while I admired them. Some men, he confided, wore their own Jockey shorts and stuck a pad down the front of the crotch, but there was always a potential for embarrassment. "A lot of thought went into this stuff," John said, "so why not use it, right?"

Right. I bought a couple of packages of all three products, then added disposable leakproof pads in two sizes, a couple of urinals, and three medical sheepskins, which John promised would make sitting much more comfortable. John and I packed my purchases into the car. I tried to imagine what it was actually going to be like *using* these products, but I couldn't. A lot of men went through surgery for prostate cancer without incontinence, didn't they? I said hopefully to John. Absolutely! he agreed heartily, but I could see from his expression that he didn't believe a word of it. I shouldn't worry, he told me. He would keep a good stock of Depends in my size, just in case.

When I got home, I sat down in the kitchen and poured myself a cup of coffee. For the first time since I had received the news that I had cancer, I felt like crying. It was dawning on me just how different my life would be after the twenty-ninth, perhaps not forever, to be sure, but for a long time. I would have to learn to live with incontinence, even if it was short-lived. I could expect to be impotent for the best part of a year. Judging from the mimeographed sheet that Dr. Walsh offered his patients, I would not be able to drink caffeinated beverages, anything carbonated, or any kind of alcohol, including wine, all of which would make it more difficult to regain continence, as well as making the incontinence worse.

No wine, no sex, no coffee, and a closet full of incontinence products! I sipped my coffee and gave myself permission to feel self-pity. And why not? A stiff upper lip is fine for facing the outside world, but you can't keep it stiff twenty-four hours a day, least of all with yourself. Every once in a while, it does no harm to feel sorry for yourself—if nothing else, cancer should permit that. It sometimes helps to admit that you're scared.

I admitted it to myself, and to Margaret, on the way down to Baltimore, as we reread the instructions Dr. Walsh's office had mailed me.

12

My operation was scheduled for the morning of Tuesday, November 29, but I was required to be at Johns Hopkins for registration and "pre-op" at two in the afternoon the day before, a process which, I had been advised, would take "several hours." I was to make no plans for the evening—not that I could imagine taking advantage of Baltimore's nightlife the night before Dr. Walsh was to operate on me.

I would not spend Monday night, before the operation, in the hospital—the insurance companies have seen to it that everybody's hospital stay is reduced to the absolute minimum. Instead, I was to arrive at Johns Hopkins at seven A.M. on Tuesday, with all my things. I would proceed directly to the surgical wing and would not see my hospital room until I was moved to it from the Intensive Care Unit, after surgery. From Monday lunchtime on I was restricted to liquids—water, cranberry juice (orange juice, you may be interested to know, counts as a solid, as does yogurt), or Jell-O. Before midnight I was to give myself a Fleet enema, with which I would be provided, and I would give myself another in the morning. After midnight I was to drink nothing at all. If I was thirsty, I could rub an ice cube on my lips.

My level of anxiety can be judged by the fact that I had an episode of fear and rage on Saturday, a kind of mini–nervous breakdown, when I—normally the best-organized of people—became somehow convinced that I had mixed the dates up and that we should already have been on our way to Baltimore; on top of which, I couldn't find the tickets. I ended up with all my neatly arranged files scattered over my study floor, trembling, howling, tears pouring down my cheeks, while Margaret held me in her arms and tried to calm me down. Of course I was wrong about the date, and of course the tickets turned up, but this was merely the pretext for my outburst. I had been waiting, it seemed endlessly, for the moment of truth, and now that it was inescapably close, I was terrified of it.

All of Margaret's concerns about how I would manage to get home *from* Baltimore were borne out by our flight *to* it. We experienced every possible inconvenience of air travel: traffic jams threatened to make us late for our flight; there was confusion and chaos at La Guardia, where construction is apparently under way forever; our flight to Pittsburgh was delayed; and when we arrived there it was only to face another inexplicable (and unexplained) delay of several hours in the flight to Baltimore, where we finally arrived near midnight, exhausted and starving, no food having been served on the way. The journey had proved Margaret right. Even *I* couldn't imagine how I would deal with all that on the way back home six or seven days after surgery, wearing a Foley catheter and a leg bag for urine.

We arrived at the hotel with an astonishing amount of luggage, most of it mine. In Margaret's case that was understandable, since all sorts of friends were proposing to come down to give her company and sympathy and take her out to dinner. Dick Snyder, my old friend and ex-boss, had booked a room; Rod Barker, an author and dear friend, was flying all the way from New Mexico; Avi Offit and her husband, Sidney, planned to come down when I had recovered enough to appreciate company. . . . In my own case, there was less excuse for all my luggage, heavy with books, laptop, envelopes full of work to catch up on. (All I would really need, it turned out, was a robe, slippers, a toothbrush, and an electric razor.)

We ate the ritual Baltimore crab cakes in our suite, watched an old movie on television, and slept uneasily in each other's arms. Always the congenital optimist (and overachiever), I had brought my running shoes and a sweatsuit with me, planning to take a run in the morning, but when I woke up it was pouring rain, a dismal, dark day, and my mood was in concert with the weather, so I decided that my cardiovascular system would have to look after itself for once. I let Margaret sleep late, then we ate breakfast and went downstairs to look at our watches and kill time. Neither of us was hungry, but eating seemed a way of using up time, which, by now, was beginning to weigh heavily on us. We sat down in one of the hotel's restaurants for lunch. Margaret picked at her food, and I ate a cup of chicken consommé and a bowl of Jell-O, trying hard to pretend that this was a normal meal, until we could finally go to the lobby and ask the doorman to get us a taxi.

Where to? he asked. Johns Hopkins, I said. He nodded knowingly. One look at us was enough to tell him which one of us was the patient—probably a significant number of the hotel's guests came here only because Johns Hopkins was fifteen minutes away. He had seen it all before.

"Good luck," he said mournfully, like a man saying good-bye to a prisoner on his way to the guillotine, and he shook my hand solemnly before opening the passenger door, promising to make sure Margaret got a taxi every morning.

—◆—

ON MY LAST visit to Johns Hopkins, four weeks before, I had been seeking answers to my questions. It had not seemed a threatening place, nor had I felt myself to be a part of it—I was a visitor, due to go back home to New York the same day. This time, I was about to become a patient; the endless, unimaginable resources of one of the world's great hospitals would soon be concentrated on me. I felt much as I had done as I passed through the gates of a new school, or standing in my civilian clothes with my suitcase in front of the guardhouse for recruit training. I would not be here as long as the time I had passed in those other institutions, but the feeling was the same, the sense of being "a new boy," with a new set of rules and rituals to learn, and unfamiliar orders to obey.

The afternoon had the "hurry up and wait" pace of the armed forces, together with the endless bureaucratic form-filling that hospitals and the military share. As Margaret and I made our way from office to office, I would not have been surprised if someone had shoved a stack of uniforms toward me over a counter—except for my orange plastic Johns Hopkins patient identification card, I might as well have been a recruit. Eventually, we completed our obstacle course through the business office—I had speeded up the process as much as I could by faxing all the information they needed in advance, something I strongly recommend doing with any hospital. My blood was taken, for the umpteenth time, my papers and charts checked, my living will clipped into my folder in case it was needed, then we went upstairs for a full physical for me, after which we were told to wait in the Marburg Building, where Dr. Walsh, or one of his assistants, would brief us on what to expect the following day. On no account were we to stray, for by now I was entered on the computer as one of the patients Dr. Walsh would operate on the next morning ("How many does he do in one day?" Margaret asked), and my whereabouts were suddenly everybody's concern.

Johns Hopkins is so huge that the journey from where we were to "Marburg," as everyone calls Dr. Walsh's domain, seemed to take forever. We took stairs, people movers, escalators, and elevators, following signposts through corridors packed with nurses and doctors and finally emerging into a small, dim, sparsely furnished waiting room. A nurse appeared, checked my name off on her list, and asked us to sit down and wait. Up until then I had been fairly cheerful, or at least resigned, perhaps because I had something to do, even if it was only trying to arrive promptly at the next appointment on our list. Now, suddenly, it was almost early evening, and I felt exhausted. Marburg was where I would be tomorrow, after I came up from the ICU—one of these rooms would be mine. I glanced down the corridor. A bent-over figure in a checked bathrobe was shuffling up and down in his slippered feet, pushing an IV stand before him. Plastic tubes attached him to what seemed to be a small computer. His progress was slow and not particularly steady. Bells pinged loudly through the ward. I felt like an interloper.

I sat down next to Margaret and held her hand. A bell rang and the elevator doors opened. Two attendants wheeled out a bed bearing a middle-aged man attached to monitors and IV units. He gave a weak thumbs-up sign as he was moved past us toward his room. His face, under the sparse neon light, was the color of cream cheese, but with a slight bluish tint. "Oh, God!" I said.

Margaret squeezed my hand hard. "You're going to be okay," she said firmly.

"That's going to be me tomorrow."

"Well, he looked all right, didn't he?"

"He looked like death warmed over. And what were those blue things wrapped around his legs for?" The man's legs had been encased in what looked like bulky gaiters, or the kind of protective wraps that are put around horses' legs to ship them. These were attached to a small machine that made a soft, slow, breathing noise.

"I don't know, but I'm sure we'll find out."

"I wish I hadn't seen him."

"He was well enough to give you a thumbs-up sign. I'll bet you do, too."

I wasn't so sure. Warm as it was in the waiting area, the sight of the man being wheeled toward his room after surgery had chilled me to the bone. I had an inkling of what it must feel like to be a condemned man, the feeling of being trapped, committed to a fate over which I had no control. Of course, it wasn't true. I could have walked out of the hospital and taken the next train back to New York, but I knew I wasn't going to do that.

Eventually, another couple arrived, looking apprehensive and a little rattled, he clutching a manila envelope identical to mine—clearly he was a fellow patient. We introduced ourselves. Ned and Gladys Mynatt were from Tennessee, and had, as I am sure we did, the look of people at the end of their tether. Ned and I exchanged PSA levels and Gleason scores companionably. His were about the same as mine, and he, too, had immediately decided on their meeting that Dr. Walsh was his man.

Ned was soft-spoken, courtly, and a little shy; Gladys, more out-going. Ned was going first in the morning, before me. I wondered which was better. Did Dr. Walsh need "warming up," like an athlete, or was he fresh for the first operation of the morning, then tired for the next one? Ned and I batted this one around to pass the time, but his heart wasn't in it. His eyes were wide open, like those of an animal trapped in oncoming headlights, while Gladys and Margaret chatted quietly in a corner. The reason for our wait, Ned told me, was that a *third* patient was expected, who was being operated on by one of Dr. Walsh's colleagues. His plane was delayed by bad weather (during the course of the afternoon at Johns Hopkins I had forgotten that in the outside world it had been pouring rain), and since nobody wanted to waste time going through the familiarization process twice, we were to sit here until he arrived. I made an expedition to the cafeteria, and came back with a bottle of apple juice, since I was beginning to feel famished.

I offered some to Ned, but he shook his head. "How do you feel about all this?" he asked.

"Scared," I said. "That, and I'd like to get it over, for better or worse. The waiting is a killer."

It was not the happiest choice of words, but Ned nodded. "Me too," he said.

I asked Ned how he was planning to get home after the surgery, and learned that he and Gladys were simply going to fly back the way they'd come, which Dr. Walsh had assured them would be fine. Ned asked me if I had made arrangements with my local urologist to have my catheter removed three weeks after surgery, which Dr. Walsh had asked him to do. I had not even *thought* about it, and realized suddenly that for all my laying in of supplies and making contact with the local nursing services, I had no urologist in Dutchess County, where I would be recuperating. If I had a problem, I was hardly likely to want to go all the way down to New York City to consult a urologist. Wondering what else I had forgotten to do, I asked Margaret to call a doctor neighbor of ours and ask him for a recommendation.

I liked Ned instantly. He had the kind of instant friendliness that is so common outside New York City and Los Angeles, and so rare in them. He was still having trouble convincing himself that he was really there, in Johns Hopkins, about to go under the knife. He had felt fine—he *still* felt fine, come to that. There had been no symptoms, no advance warning of any kind. He had never even *thought* about his prostate, which, unlike mine, had not given him a bit of trouble, ever, and so had been unprepared for the grim tone in his urologist's voice when he called to say that Ned's PSA was elevated.

The long wait in a small, dark space at the end of a hospital corridor, facing the elevator, was rapidly raising our collective anxiety level. I felt like one of the characters in Sartre's *No Exit,* condemned to spend the rest of eternity in a small room with three other people. From time to time, a nurse would appear to announce that Dr. Walsh would be with us "soon." Eventually, she reappeared to announce that the chief resident would be talking to us instead of Dr. Walsh, and that we would first hear from the head surgical nurse, as soon as she arrived. In the meantime, she handed us a stack of things to read. Most of them were forms advising us of our rights as patients, others warned of dire consequences for such things as taking aspirin. Luckily for me, Dr. Walsh had made it very clear that I must not take aspirin in the weeks preceding the surgery, since it promotes bleeding. Others, I discovered, had not been so well informed. One man I talked to had arrived for his operation (not at Johns Hopkins) and was asked, just as he was being wheeled down to the operating room, whether he had been taking aspirin. He replied that he had, and was wheeled right back again, given his street clothes, and sent home to wait four weeks before he could be operated on. Nobody had told him about aspirin. Another lesson, I thought: Always ask questions, however obvious they may seem, and do not assume that the doctor will think of everything.

At last, the head nurse appeared, even though the missing patient had not. She ran through what was facing us tomorrow. We were to check in at the business office and proceed directly to the surgical wing—she passed out maps. We should bring our suitcases, which would be moved into our rooms. After we had undressed and put on hospital gowns; we would receive IVs in the arm; then, at the appropriate moment, the anesthesiologist would insert an epidural. This epidural would serve as the conduit for the anesthetic before and during the operation, and for the painkiller afterward. Glasses, watches, and so forth, we should make sure to hand to our spouses. Were there any questions?

I raised my hand. I was deathly afraid of having an epidural, I said. Would it be painful? The nurse shook her head. I wouldn't feel a thing, she assured me. I should mention my anxiety to the anesthesiologist, who would probably give me Valium. She made a note on her clipboard.

When we woke up in the recovery unit, she continued, we would find our legs enclosed in special compression hose—she held up a shiny white stocking with a hole for the big toe. On top of these would be a bulkier leg covering hitched up to a compression device that would gently "pump" the legs at regular intervals, to keep the circulation moving and prevent embolism. These were the sky-blue leg wrappings I had seen on the patient who gave us the thumbs-up sign as he emerged from the elevator. We would be attached to the compression device for about twenty-four hours. The support hose we would wear for the next four weeks, and before we left the hospital we would be shown how to put them on.

We would also be taught how to care for the Foley catheter which was to be our closest companion for the next three weeks or so. We would have a regular bag—she held one up, and it looked like a deflated balloon—and a leg bag for walking about—she held up a small, rectangular plastic pouch with tubes at either end and two Velcro straps that were designed to be tightened around the thigh and just below the knee. Did we have any questions?

I had plenty, but nothing that I wanted to bring up here. How would I feel when I woke up in the recovery room? How much pain would I experience? What would the catheter feel like? What would *I* feel like when I was lying in the operating room, and once again, would it hurt when they put the epidural in? Instead, Ned and I shook our heads in unison, as if we knew everything we wanted to know.

The elevator door opened and a tall, bulky, red-faced man, built along the lines of Falstaff, emerged with his wife in tow. Bob Smith was from South Carolina, with the big, hearty voice and eager hand-shake that Easterners wrongly assume is a Texas hallmark, and he swiftly filled the room with his presence. Gail Smith was small, pretty, and blond, considerably younger than her husband, and dressed to the nines. Their plane had been delayed, and their bag-gage had been lost. Bob had been afraid he wasn't going to make it, he boomed, as if he was late for a party, but here he was, rarin' to go. He exuded solid good-fellowship, and seemed bigger—or perhaps more cheerful—than life, possibly because unlike the rest of us he hadn't been cooped up in a small airless room for hours—waiting for him, as a matter of fact. There was a slight undertow of resent-ment at his presence, now that he had finally turned up. A close look, however, revealed that underneath the bluster Bob was as scared as Ned and I.

At least he was frank about it, which was more than could be said of me. "Ah'm scared, fellows," he announced. As if his having cancer wasn't enough, his doctor had refused to perform surgery on him un-less he lost weight, so he had been on a crash diet and dropped twenty-four pounds. Shortly, we knew all about him. He was a busi-nessman who raised cattle on the side, and he still couldn't believe that any of this was happening to him. I could tell that he took it per-sonally, as if somebody must be responsible for this major fuckup and would have to answer the consequences. There was something about his honest, uncomplicated expression of fear and his need for reassurance that made Ned and me feel like pillars of stability, as op-posed to the quaking mounds of Jell-O we knew ourselves to be on the inside. There is nothing like being drawn into someone else's dis-tress to relieve one's own.

Ned and I filled Bob in, like old cons greeting a new prisoner, while Margaret and Gladys conferred with Gail about her missing baggage. Bob, too, was an innocent when it came to hospitals, and so far wasn't enjoying the experience a bit. He had been rushing from one office to another, desperately trying to get all his papers in order, while everywhere he went loudspeakers called him urgently to the Marburg Pavilion. His face was beet-red with exertion, and it looked as if he might actually need a cardiologist before he ever got into the hands of a urologist.

A nurse arrived to confirm that Bob had shown up. She brandished a piece of paper. If we wanted television, she said, we must be sure to sign up for it tomorrow morning when we arrived at the hospital, or it would not be activated by the time we got to our rooms. Television was the last thing on my mind, but for some reason, Margaret was convinced I must have it. She would take care of it herself, she promised me, grabbing the form from the nurse as if my life depended on it.

What seemed like an age passed, and finally, a real, live *doctor* appeared, dressed in surgical greens and looking even more exhausted than we were. He introduced himself.

The chief resident had the look of a football coach as he leaned against a pillar to prep us for the coming day's game plan. He had a pleasant Hispanic accent and an easy, engaging smile. We were to make sure that we had all our papers with us—the bureaucracy had to be served. If we had made out a living will it must be clipped into the surgeon's files. He reminded us that we were on a liquid diet, and that by "liquid" he did *not* mean alcoholic beverages. From midnight on, we were to take nothing. If we were thirsty, we could touch an ice cube to our lips. He reminded us sternly about our Fleet enemas. Tomorrow morning, at the appointed time, each of us would meet up with his anesthesiologists while waiting to be taken to the operating room. Each of us would have an IV placed in his wrist. After that, the anesthesiologists (at Johns Hopkins they apparently traveled in packs) would take us into Dr. Walsh's operating room and insert an epidural. In Bob's case, the procedure would be a little different, since his surgeon, unlike Dr. Walsh, used a full general anesthetic.

I looked at Bob with some envy. That Bob would be out cold—as dead to the world as a steer that had just been poleaxed—seemed like a better way to go. The doctor didn't agree, though. He felt that there was not a lot of difference between the two approaches. The epidural was perhaps a fraction safer, and the patient might recover from it a little more quickly, but in either case, none of us would feel anything. He himself—not surprisingly—agreed with Dr. Walsh that the epidural was a superior procedure for this operation. He, too, showed us the anti-embolism devices we would be wearing on our legs when we awoke in the recovery room. We should also expect to have a drain, to one side of the incision in the abdomen. This would have a bulb on it, so that the fluids and blood seepage could be removed at regular intervals. We would keep the drain for five days, and it would be removed before we left the hospital, along with the staples in the incision. Both procedures were quick and not at all painful.

We would be served our first meal the day after surgery. It was *not* optional. We must eat all of it, hungry or not. It was vitally important to get the digestive system functioning again after major surgery, and we would not be able to leave the hospital until we had experienced our first bowel movement. Gas pains might be a problem, although the gas was, of itself, a good sign rather than a bad one. We should report gas pain to the nurses—it could be alleviated. However, the sooner we were up and walking about, the sooner the gas would pass. And the sooner we had a full bowel movement, the sooner we could start thinking about home. Were there any questions?

I raised my hand and explained again about my fear of epidurals.

He nodded encouragingly—or perhaps patiently, as one might humor a mild lunatic. There was nothing to be afraid of, he said firmly. I would be given Valium before the epidural catheter was inserted. I wouldn't even know it was happening. At most I would feel a mild sting.

I thanked him, but my stomach was churning. "A mild sting" sounds okay, but coming from the lips of a surgeon, who could say what that really meant?

He looked at his watch, and dismissed us. "Get a good night's sleep," he said, as if that were possible. We would see him again when we were safely in our rooms after surgery.

"*Hasta la vista,* baby," I heard one of our party murmur, in imitation of Arnold Schwarzenegger, but it fell flat. Nobody was in a laughing mood.

———————

THAT NIGHT MARGARET and I ordered room service, the usual Maryland crab cakes for her, a bottle of mineral water for me. We sat and chatted until the table had been taken away, then went to bed, and lay there, side by side, reading our books and holding hands. Margaret and I have always found hotel rooms sexy, perhaps because so much of our relationship was spent in them when we were having an affair and still married to other people. Or maybe everybody finds hotel rooms sexy, who knows?

Anyway, we stuffed ourselves with sleeping pills (there was no preoperative prohibition against them), turned the lights off, and made love, in a strange, almost passionless way, for the truth was that neither one of us was much aroused—the anxiety level was simply too high for that. I could not help wondering if this was going to be the last time I ever performed this familiar act which had played so large a part in my life since adolescence, and which indeed had often seemed like the center of life, the only part of it that made sense. At the very least it would never *feel* like this again, I knew, feeling the familiar excitement of ejaculation, the spurt of semen, the deep peace that comes with orgasm and the feel of one's own body liquids.

Whatever was going to happen to me, the discharge of semen and seminal fluids would never be a part of my life again. Perhaps that wasn't such a big deal, I told myself. Worse things could surely happen, and probably would, in time. But somehow the reality of sex is fluid, liquid, wet, as every pornographer knows—it is no accident that an ability to ejaculate copiously is almost as important a qualification for porn movie stardom as penis size, as we learn from Richard Rhodes's *Making Love.* Intercourse is a messy business—that is part of its pleasure, after all.

I felt like crying, but I knew that would do no good and would simply upset Margaret, whose control over herself was fragile at that moment, so we did what we could, then held hands under the sheets and waited for the sleeping pills to work. "Thank you," I said, kissing Margaret's shoulder, but she was already dozing uneasily, so I set aside her book and closed my eyes.

But I had much to thank her for, not the least of which was that I would remember this night as vividly as the most passionate nights of our lives, when we were still lovers new to each other, weaving complicated and unlikely scenarios that would enable us to spend a rare night together.

The night in Baltimore lacked that kind of excitement, to be sure, but I will remember every detail of it with profound emotion for the rest of my life—though, of course, I didn't know that at the time, which was probably just as well.

I went to sleep at last, and woke up in the early morning, as afraid of my epidural as I had ever been.

13

TUESDAY WAS GRAY AND GRIM. I FELT CURIOUS—HUNGRY, THIRSTY, and completely well. It seemed like a mistake to subject this seemingly healthy body to surgery. Would I ever wake up feeling this good again? I wondered. To end *that* kind of thinking, I made my way to the bathroom and gave myself a final Fleet enema, rather proud that I was getting pretty good at it by now.

If there is a less attractive way of starting a day than lying on the marble floor of a hotel bathroom in the exact posture of the androgynous model pictured on a Fleet enema package, I don't know what it is. I had a schoolboy horror of being sent home in disgrace by Dr. Walsh because I hadn't managed to get my colon clean enough (it *does* happen), so I tried to hold in the liquid for as long as possible, no easy or comfortable task, since the colder a Fleet enema is, the better it works, and this one was really *chilly.* On my side, knees drawn up, the contents of the Fleet enema squeezed into my rectum, I clenched my sphincter muscles as hard as I could and tried to read *The New York Times.* When I couldn't hold it in anymore, I crawled clumsily to the toilet, and hoped Dr. Walsh would be satisfied. I certainly was. I felt cleansed and empty as never before.

I finished *The New York Times,* ordered Margaret's breakfast, shaved, brushed my teeth (thinking, all the time, Does any of this matter?), bathed. I would be, if nothing else, the cleanest person Dr. Walsh had ever operated on. I remembered the story about Harold Lear, a distinguished urologist, in Martha Lear's book *Heartsounds.* Dr. Lear said that when a patient called him with a problem, he always advised him to take a long, hot bath. Did that help? a student asked him. No, Lear replied, but at least when the patient came to his office the next day he was clean!

We dressed, and went downstairs to kill time in the hotel lobby. I kept looking at my watch, wondering if I had forgotten to wind it. Finally it was time to perform a last, small ritual. I handed Margaret my watch, my briefcase with all my papers in it, my wallet, my keys, and my credit cards. "You're going to be in the driver's seat for a while now," I said jokingly.

Margaret nodded. She did not laugh. She would be in the driver's seat, as it turned out, for longer than either of us imagined, but although she did splendidly at it, she didn't like it a bit.

I took my bag, heavy with what I thought of as hospital necessities, and we set off for Johns Hopkins, hand in hand, in silence.

By now, I thought, my friends Ned and Bob were already being operated on.

———✠———

IN THE CAVERNOUS halls of Johns Hopkins we went through the familiar process of form-filling, blood test (why? I asked myself; surely by now they must know everything there is to know about my blood), waiting in line, and moving from floor to floor. We were, naturally, earlier than we needed to be, but even so the time got used up, and I had ample opportunities to say the word *cancer* when asked what I was there for, though by now it was second nature, as easy as saying my name or remembering my Social Security number.

Just before we were about to enter the elevator that would take us to the operating rooms, Margaret remembered my television service, and went off to pay for it in advance. I could see that for some reason this was important to her, that she wanted me to take it seriously and show gratitude for her concern; then it occurred to me that television, of course, represented *normality,* life as usual—that if, as she told me, I would not want to miss *NYPD Blue* or *ER,* it was because my desire not to miss them would be a sign I was well, recovering, able to focus on the things that were familiar to us.

Still, television was the last thing on my mind as we got into the elevator—a large one, ominously suitable for a gurney—and made our way to a tiny, cramped waiting room in the surgical area, packed with miserable and unhappy people. Some of the people waiting to be called for surgery were accompanied by their whole families, including aged grandmothers muttering prayers, bulky gold-chained uncles, muscular teenaged boys in team sweatshirts, sultry-looking teenaged girls plastered in makeup. There was a boy waiting to have surgery on his knee, accompanied by his football teammates, all of them as noisy and cheerful as if this were a party.

It was hot in the room, the animal warmth adding itself to suffocating central heating and the presence of many heavy winter coats, but there was no way out. At one end was the elevator, at the other, the door that led to pre-op—it might have been the anteroom to hell.

I decided that the only way to survive was to read my way through it. I took out a volume of A.J.P. Taylor's essays on nineteenth-century European history and plunged into Bismarckian diplomacy. Time passed, slowly; then, after the room had pretty much emptied out, a nurse appeared and called us in.

"What next?" Margaret whispered as we were shown into a big room separated by curtains into bed-sized cubicles, one of which was mine.

I shook my head. I had no idea. There were two chairs, and we sat.

"How are you feeling?" Margaret asked.

I said I was okay. It was true, but fear was beginning to grow inside me. Waiting, I realized, was the thing that made it happen, but waiting was an intrinsic part of the process. I hoped my courage—or whatever it was that was holding me together—would last until they took me away.

Eventually, an intern came by and we started to get down to business. My file was produced, we verified that my living will was stapled to the file cover, we went over all the forms to make sure that I was the right person—a sensible precaution in a large hospital—then I was handed another form, which already bore Dr. Walsh's signature, in which I was to confirm that I had been warned the operation might have as its consequences death, impotence, and/or incontinence, and that it had been explained to me that alternative treatments included radiation, hormone therapy, or watchful waiting, and that I had rejected them. I signed with a flourish. By now I was anxious to get it all done with.

"I'm really afraid of the epidural," I told the intern, an earnest young man who seemed to have picked up his bedside manner from young Mr. Carter, the intern in *ER*. Interns, as I was soon to discover, might not *know* much, but they were generally a lot more patient than their seniors. "I just have this *block* about spinal taps," I told him.

He consulted the file. "Yes," he said, "there's a note about it here. Listen, it's nothing, but I'll get the anesthesiologist to talk to you about it as soon as he has time. Now get undressed and put on your gown. Your clothes will go up to your room."

I got undressed and slipped into the shapeless, limp cotton gown, beginning to feel chilled and more vulnerable now that my clothes, the last things that separated me from being "a patient," had been removed. I had been given paper slippers. I put them on, too, then sat down, feeling miserably sorry for myself at last.

Soon, however, an agreeable young nurse arrived and inserted the IV drip into my wrist. I was now attached to a saline drip bag on a chrome pole, with wheels so I could push it around. A plastic hospital ID tag was fastened to my other wrist. We were getting somewhere now. I told her about my fear of epidurals. She told me not to worry about it.

I asked when I would be shaved. She laughed. "Not until you're out," she said. "It's easier that way."

Margaret and I sat quietly while my IV line dripped. On the other side of the curtain separating us from the next cubicle a husband was saying good-bye to his wife, who was awaiting surgery. Their three small children cried and quarreled while she made him recite all the things he had to do to look after them.

"I'd drown them on my way home," Margaret said through clenched teeth. Every once in a while one of the kids would stick his head under the curtain into my cubicle and make a face at us. I made one back, eventually, and he burst into tears.

The head nurse appeared to inform us that I would be going shortly. After I had once more shared my fear of epidurals, I asked her if I could go to the bathroom.

She raised an eyebrow. "The bathroom? They may be coming for you any moment."

"I need to urinate. I don't see why I should have to go into surgery on a full bladder."

This was apparently not a part of the routine. I pushed my IV pole on its little wheels down the corridor, and peed normally, for the last time, I realized, for many, many months. When I got back to the cubicle, the woman next to me had gone. I relished the quiet, but in a moment the curtain was pulled back and two handsome, cheerful young men in pale-blue scrub suits appeared, grinning. "Are you the guy who's afraid of epidurals?" the older of the two asked.

I said I was, and repeated my whole spinal tap number.

He consulted his clipboard. "Got it," he said. "We're your anesthesiology team. It says right here: patient expresses fears about epidural. You want it from the horse's mouth? The way I do it you won't feel a thing. Okay?"

"Not okay," I said. "I don't believe you."

"Scout's honor. Nobody complains. Tell you what, I'll give you so much Valium you won't even feel it go in."

I nodded. Maybe it was the IV drip, but I was beginning to feel more relaxed. "When do we start?" I asked.

"Right now," they said. The older doctor glanced at his chart again. "We can sedate you deeply, you know, or keep you conscious enough so that you can watch the operation. That's the beauty of an epidural. You won't *feel* anything, but you'll be able to see what's going on. It's up to you."

"I'd rather be out like a light, please. I don't want to see a thing, or even *remember* a thing."

He scribbled a quick note to himself. "You got it. You're going to miss a pretty interesting piece of surgery, but it's your call. Better kiss your wife good-bye."

I kissed Margaret, handed her my eyeglasses, and told her to make sure she got something for lunch. Then they hustled me into a wheelchair, out of her sight, and pushed me swiftly down a long hallway and through a swinging door into Dr. Walsh's operating room.

My first impression was that it was small, cramped, and dark. I had been expecting a brightly lit operating theater, but this was nothing like that. There was a silver-colored operating table with a kind of long armrest—or was it a backrest?—built into it. On the right was a huge mass of electronic black boxes, clearly the equipment for the anesthesiologists; on the left was a big chrome table with all Dr. Walsh's instruments laid out in a neat, shiny row. I don't know whether Dr. Walsh was in the room, but I had a vague impression that there was a group of people in surgical scrubs standing in the shadows, chatting.

I was asked to lean forward against the armrest, or shelf, or whatever it was, exposing my back. The moment for the dreaded epidural had arrived. "I'm not usually like this," I said to the anesthesiologist as he gave me an injection. "I mean, I've seen some pretty bad things in my time, medically speaking. I was in the hospital in Budapest, in '56, during the revolution, and saw them operating on the wounded without any kind of anesthesia because they had run out . . . amputations, stomach wounds, you name it. . . ."

"That must have been something," he said, with the voice of a doctor humoring a patient. It occurred to me that he probably wasn't even *born* in '56, and probably had never heard of the '56 uprising.

"What I mean is that I'm not *squeamish,*" I explained carefully. "It's just that I have this irrational fear about epidurals."

"I know," he said. "It's in your folder."

"When is it going in?" I asked.

"It's already in," he said, and that was the last thing I remember until I came to in the recovery room a few hours later.

14

SIX MONTHS AFTER SURGERY I TOOK TO LUNCH A LITERARY AGENT who is well known for her practice of leaking whatever she's told to the press—a bad habit which normally makes me reticent in her presence. When she asked me about my surgery, however, I opened up—six months after surgery it's rare to be with somebody to whom one hasn't already told the story at least once, so a new listener is always welcome. It was a mistake, of course. The very next morning a reporter from the *New York Observer* called me to ask if it was true that I had had a "near death" experience. I assured him that it was not, with some annoyance, but on later reflection it occurred to me that perhaps, in fact, I *had*.

Recovering from the anesthesia was as close to "near death" as I ever want to come. I was dimly aware of light, of movement, of motions around me, but I couldn't *focus* on them, as if I were being drawn back into unconsciousness, a sensation like drowning, but without any physical struggle, shortness of breath, or panic—a *peaceful* drowning, if there is such a thing.

I don't know how long the sensation lasted, but it gradually dawned on me that the motion around me was coming not, as I had at first assumed, from the spirit world, but from my own. My vision was blurred, but I could tell that nurses were working around me, and could feel, just as promised, a gentle pumping action on my swaddled legs. I thought I saw Margaret, and wondered how she had got there—wherever "there" was—before me. "Am I alive?" I croaked, surprised at how hard it was to make a sound.

"Of course you are," she said, stroking my hand gently.

I was quietly pleased. Professor Martin, I recalled, had been advised to feel for the catheter emerging from his penis. Its presence would confirm that the operation had been completed—that, in other words, the surgeon had *not* found cancer in the lymph nodes or the surrounding tissue, but I could not bring myself to touch anything down there. I could feel the presence of numerous tubes, dressings, and staples, and assumed all was well. I really didn't care much, one way or the other, and simply wanted to be left alone.

Of course, that's the one thing that isn't going to happen in a hospital after major surgery. People kept appearing in my line of sight to ask me how I felt, but I could only mumble. Somebody put a piece of ice on my lips. At intervals, the bag for my IV was replaced as it emptied. Eventually, I fell back into a kind of sweaty doze, not quite awake, not quite asleep, lulled by the rhythmic chug and click of the machine that was pumping my legs. I, who am normally so busy, had nowhere to go and nothing I needed to do. I felt strangely relaxed and free of obligations. Whatever was going on, for the moment no effort was required of me except to keep breathing, rather like a baby in its crib. It was a not unpleasant sensation.

Time passed. I felt a rocking motion, more movement, then I opened my eyes again and I found myself in another room, surrounded by flowers, as if I really *were* dead this time. I saw Margaret looking down at me, and said, "Hello, I love you, I'm alive." "Me too," she said. "Now shush." She squeezed my hand, and I dozed again.

—m—

WHEN I WOKE up again I was in a hospital room. To my left was a bedside table and my IV unit. To my right, a thick bundle of wires and tubes, as well as a couple of plastic bulbs about the size of softballs, full of bloody liquid—my drains were apparently functioning as they were intended to. There was a window that looked out on a stone wall, a television set bolted to a metal rack, and enough flowers for a gangster funeral.

"How do you feel?" I heard Margaret ask.

"Awful," I said. It wasn't so much a question of pain as of intense unease, as if whole areas of my body were coming back to life and trying to make me aware that something terrible had happened. I reminded myself that just a few hours ago I had felt perfectly well. It was a depressing thought.

"Lie still," Margaret said, but lying still was all I could do, the focus, as it happened, of all my concentration.

Time passed. I held on to Margaret's hand. From time to time, more flowers arrived, and she read the names on the cards to me. "You're feeling very hot," she said. "Are you all right?"

I thought that was odd. Truth to tell, I was feeling so cold that my teeth were chattering. "Close the window," I managed to say, but the window *was* closed—in fact, Margaret pointed out, the room was stifling.

A nurse bent over to check my urine bag—I had managed to locate the Foley catheter by now. More flowers arrived: a huge display of white roses. The nurse paused to admire them. I felt a strange, sinking sensation, separate from the extreme cold. It was, I imagine, what hypothermia must feel like, when people die from extreme cold and severe exposure, a slow drift toward a peaceful end. I really had no sensation at all, except for the numbing chill.

I was aware of a bustle of activity. Margaret had grabbed the nurse, and directed her attention away from the flowers and toward me. "I don't like the way he looks," she said. "His face is as white as a sheet. His *lips and fingernails* are as white as a sheet, for God's sake! Feel his face. He's burning up!"

I felt a tightening on my arm as my blood pressure was taken. In fact, though I was, perhaps fortunately, unaware of it, this was a difficult moment, since the nurse had neglected to attach the tube from the cuff to the measuring device and was unable to produce a reading. As soon as Margaret pointed out the problem, things started to happen in a hurry. More nurses arrived, then doctors—interns, at first, then the resident, all in their green scrubs, then a senior doctor in a white coat. What had happened, I was later to discover, was that I had suffered a precipitous drop in blood pressure, not uncommon after this kind of surgery but no less frightening for that. Since two of the three pints of blood I had donated autologously had been used up during the actual surgery, I had only one pint left. It was brought from whatever far recesses of the hospital blood was stored in and attached to my IV. I remember looking up at the bag of blood with a kind of detached interest, noticing how slowly the level went down—very different from the speed with which it had filled up when I donated the blood. This, it turned out, was a problem. The blood had come straight from storage—it was cold, and therefore viscous and slow-flowing, so it took a long time to get it into my system. A second problem was that it made me feel even colder. I had every blanket on top of me, plus my bathrobe—a habit I was not to give up for months—and still I shivered and chattered my teeth.

And yet, I was alert again, and able to understand what had happened to me—once someone explained it. That, I thought, was a good sign. The dying aren't interested in explanations, nor does anybody feel the need to explain things to them. Pain was beginning to bother me. I complained about it.

The doctor in the white coat nodded. He didn't think the pain would get too bad, but there was a slight problem with pain medication at the moment. Painkillers lowered the blood pressure. My blood pressure was already way, way down—getting better, to be sure, but still far too low. I would have to do without painkillers until my blood pressure stabilized.

My first thought was, This can't be happening, but clearly it was. How long would I have to go without painkillers? I asked. The answer was a couple of hours, perhaps. Probably not more. It might get a little rough, but I would simply have to take it.

The phrase "bite the bullet" came to my mind. In the eighteenth and nineteenth centuries, wounded soldiers literally clamped their teeth on a lead bullet to prevent themselves from crying out in pain (civilian patients were provided with a leather strap to bite into). I had always wondered how anybody could have borne that kind of pain (not that I would compare mine to theirs), but as I was beginning to discover, when you don't have a choice about pain, you stop fighting it, and when you stop fighting it, pain becomes more bearable at once. Perhaps what makes pain terrible is the knowledge that something can be *done* about it; if it's clear that *nothing* can be done about it, the body accepts it somehow. The pain isn't *lessened;* the mind simply gives in to it. Mine did, anyway.

Now I felt warm again—sweating, in fact, with the effort of dealing with the pain, which is like hard, physical labor. It came and went in waves. "How are you doing?" Margaret whispered to me. "I wish I were dead," I said, and I was immediately sorry I had.

"You're not *ever* to say that again," Margaret said sternly.

I apologized, in a harsh, croaking whisper from my parched throat. Margaret, I realized, regarded any death wish on my part as a sign of betrayal. If I wanted to die, that signified to her that I was turning away from her, going off on my own into a world where she wouldn't be able to follow me (not for some time, at any rate). That was abandonment, in her book, and she didn't hide the fact.

—⁓—

IT WAS GETTING darker. The day was dragging to an end. Margaret left the room and came back with the local news, to distract me. Ned had come through fine, she told me, and was already sitting up and sipping on a glass of orange juice. Bob was in good shape, and already watching television, with Gail by his side. (Their luggage had reappeared, too.) He had been delighted with his full general anesthesia, and had been given morphine, which was working like a treat, for *his* pain. A more unfortunate man, across the hall from me, needed a gallbladder operation right after undergoing a radical prostatecomy, and was feeling very gloomy about life, though he, too, was watching television, or at least had it on. I could tell that Margaret felt I was letting her down by not trying out the television service after she had made sure it was activated and paid a deposit, but I simply couldn't imagine staring at the screen. The world inside my belly was the only world that was real to me for the moment.

I could hear Margaret arguing with the nurses. Apparently, pain was not in their control. Somewhere in the hospital there was a Pain Management Unit, it seemed, which was responsible for controlling pain once the patient had recovered from anesthesia. It was not clear to whom "they" reported, or where "they" were, but "they" had been beeped, and until "they" arrived nothing could be done. This was not an answer likely to satisfy Margaret, whose philosophy has always been one of instant gratification, particularly when it comes to pain relief.

From time to time as the evening progressed I heard echoes of this argument, sometimes in hushed tones close to me, sometimes more loudly in the corridor outside.

Eventually, "the pain people," as Margaret called them, turned up with their trolley, as if they were sales vendors, and examined my case. They went into a huddle. They were not so sure, it appeared, that painkillers would lower my blood pressure significantly—in any case, pain was their province, and they were not much interested in what doctors or nurses had to say about it. They were not interested in hearing from Margaret about how well Bob was doing on morphine, either. Morphine was altogether wrong for me, they said, quite out of the question, though they didn't explain why.

"Maybe they know what they're talking about," I said.

Margaret was indignant. "Of course they don't. Morphine *works.* Everybody knows that. You should see Bob. You have to insist on it."

But I was in no position to insist on anything, and besides, I assumed that the pain specialists must know what they were talking about. Argument would probably have not done any good, anyway, even if I had been up to one. The pain people's view was that of specialists the world over: nobody knew what they were talking about when it came to pain except them, and that included the patient and his doctor, not to speak of the patient's wife.

A second IV bag, containing a painkiller, was attached to my IV stand and jury-rigged to my IV tube with a little plastic valve, the flow regulated by a small computer. This was the famous "pain medication on demand" system, about which we had so often been told. A button was fastened to my hospital gown, and every time I required pain relief I could push the button, giving me an instant spurt of medication. The computer monitored the dose and was set so that I could not give myself more than one every ten minutes, but that, I was told, would be ample. I pushed the button, the computer winked, and I felt relief. It was immediate, Pavlovian. I was deeply grateful and thanked the pain people as they packed up their gear and left.

Shortly after the departure of what I now thought of as "the Pain Team," the pain came back, in waves. I pushed the button as hard as I could—and as often as I thought the computer would let me get away with—but without any effect. The nurses were sympathetic, but unhelpful, which I understood well enough by now—the pain equipment was set up, and it was not their responsibility. I was cautioned to try to take longer between doses. That didn't help, but I was reluctant to complain further, for fear of being thought a sissy— after all, I was getting the pain medication, so perhaps this level of pain was normal, though it seemed very high to me. Margaret felt otherwise. Ned, she reported, was certainly uncomfortable, but not in anything like as much pain as I was, while Bob—on morphine, of course—was "happy as a clam," watching television and making telephone calls. If *I* had insisted on morphine, she pointed out . . .

I waved this off. These people *must* know what they were doing, I said, between gasps, for by now the pain was worsening no matter how many times I pushed the damn button.

It was getting late. I wondered whether Margaret was staying past the visiting hours—not that, in her present mood, anybody was likely to evict her, for the nurses were walking on tippytoe around her by this time, eyes averted from wrath.

Soon, however, there was a noticeable increase in activity, a kind of buzz in the hive. The time was approaching for Dr. Walsh's rounds.

15

THROUGHOUT THE DAY, ANY QUESTION DIRECTED AT A NURSE—OR even a doctor—was likely to be answered with "You'll have to ask Dr. Walsh when he makes his rounds." Now the moment was approaching; all over the ward, beds were being straightened, urine bags emptied, drain pans cleaned out, patients tidied, stained hospital gowns changed. The door was open—for some reason, I was beginning to suffer from mild claustrophobia—and I could glimpse Dr. Walsh's entourage as they went from room to room, a flying wedge of green-suited doctors, with Walsh, splendid in a starched white coat over a clean shirt and businesslike tie, in the lead, as fresh and energetic as he had no doubt been at dawn, for the man seemed immune to fatigue.

He entered the room cautiously, however, having no doubt been warned that there were problems here—an unhappy patient and an angry wife. Semi-comatose as I was, I admired the doctor's control of the situation. He did not exactly *ignore* Margaret, but he concentrated his attention on me. His expression was friendly but firm, with just a hint of reproach, as if we had been making trouble. His manner suggested that if there were any misunderstandings, he was here to clear them up. First, however, he gave me the good news. I should be very happy, he said. The operation had gone splendidly. Several other doctors had observed it and been deeply impressed. He did not like to go out on a limb before the pathology report was in, which would take some time, but he had no doubt at all that he had removed all the cancer. There had been no signs of its having spread to the pelvic lymph nodes, nor beyond the prostate. He had promised me a good operation, and that was exactly what I had received.

I numbly expressed my gratitude. I should have felt elated—I *was* elated—but the day had worn me down to the point where nothing seemed to matter except what was taking place in my body. I had discovered that I felt better if I lay on my right side, with my knees drawn up slightly, as if I were cradling my tubes and drains, but it was a hard position to talk from, and it tended to cramp my right shoulder, injured in one of my innumerable riding accidents.

Margaret was describing to Dr. Walsh the events of the day, while he listened with a fixed, gentle smile. He knew all that, he seemed to be saying, but it didn't matter. What mattered was that the operation had gone perfectly, my cancer had been eliminated—*that* was what we should be concentrating on. Finally, he held his hand up, commanding silence. "Margaret," he said, his voice soft, but full of authority, "I have a protocol for wives in this hospital. The protocol is that they go back to their hotel at seven o'clock, and somebody calls them if there's a serious problem."

I closed my eyes. I heard Margaret say, in righteous anger, "I'm not leaving this hospital until my husband is comfortable and out of pain."

There was a silence. When I opened my eyes, Dr. Walsh was gone.

"I don't think we're going to be popular here," I said.

"I don't care."

A few moments later, the chief resident came in and sat down with a soft sigh. He was still dressed in his green scrubs and, unlike Dr. Walsh, showed signs of fatigue. There were deep circles under his eyes, and occasionally he rubbed them with his fists. "What seems to be the problem?" he asked.

We explained the events of the afternoon and evening. He nodded glumly. He, too, had heard it all before, from the nurses—it was probably on my chart anyway, in some abbreviated form. The pain I was complaining about in my lower abdomen was almost certainly the bladder reacting violently against the small balloon that held my Foley catheter in place, producing a sharp contraction of the bladder wall. Bladder cramps could be acutely painful. Some people got them; some didn't. Eventually, the bladder would probably get used to the presence of a foreign object inside it and settle down. Motrin helped, but since it promoted bleeding, that was out of the question for the moment. If there was no improvement by tomorrow, he would try Valium, which tended to relax the soft tissues.

As for the rest, he had reviewed my pain medication, and, really, he could find no fault in it. He would give me something to help me sleep, and if I was still uncomfortable tomorrow, he would give instructions that the Pain Management Unit should be called back.

I should try and get some sleep. Margaret, too. He appealed to her better nature—he had soft, pleading eyes, not at all like those of Dr. Walsh, which were commanding and imperious. He seemed to be trying to say, "Make my life easier, go home."

Would I feel any better?, she asked him.

He shrugged. Probably. He'd do his best. Margaret gave me a kiss and placed the TV remote where I could reach it, just in case I suddenly wanted to watch *NYPD Blue*. The doctor opened the door for her. Then he looked at me. "The first night is usually the worst," he said. "After that, it gets easier."

16

MY FRIEND KEN ARETSKY, THOUGH HE HAD TAKEN A VERY UPBEAT AT-titude toward this whole experience when he was talking me through it, had nevertheless remarked, rather casually, that he hit rock-bottom on the third morning. The *second* night, he'd said, had been the worst. After *that,* it got better. I hoped the chief resident was right, but I had more faith, really, in Ken's judgment. Surgeons don't necessarily know how it feels to be on the receiving end; patients are better judges of that.

I kept that in mind through the first night, which was, as promised, rough. The bladder cramps were intense and frequent. My bladder felt like a wild, angry animal trapped in my abdomen, trying to bite its way out. For a while it would lie still, then it would rediscover the balloon of the catheter and shy away from it violently. I lay on my right side, trying not to provoke it by moving.

From time to time a nurse appeared—a large young man, very caring and pleasant—to take my temperature and my blood pressure, check that my IV bags weren't empty, empty my catheter bag, and gently syringe out the bloody matter collected by my drains. I asked him to leave the door open. Somehow, I felt safer looking out toward the brightly lit corridor than lying alone in the dark. He looked in on me far more often than I suspected the routine was, and I was grateful. I didn't sleep. From all over the ward there was the sharp pinging noise that the IV units make when they're empty, as well as the sharper, more insistent ringing of patients buzzing for the nurse.

Dr. Walsh had made the point that he didn't allow private nurses on his ward, presumably because they got in the way of the routine, and perhaps also because he wanted a staff responsible to *him,* and trained to satisfy *his* expectations. That had made sense to me before, but I wasn't so sure now. David, the young man looking after me, could not have been nicer, but he was overwhelmed with work. I would reflect, later on, that while I never met a nurse I didn't admire and like, there were simply not enough of them—and this in one of the best and richest hospitals in the world.

By dawn, it was apparent to David (and me) that the pain medication was ineffective. He promised to alert the Pain Management Unit before he ended his shift. In the meantime, he helped me wash, gave me a plastic toothbrush and some toothpaste, and let me sip at a glass of juice. Breakfast came—I ate it slowly, feeling no hunger at all, and certainly no pleasure in the food, but conscious, having been warned, that the digestive system needed to be jump-started. The chewing wasn't so bad; it was the swallowing that was hard.

The morning brought unexpected visitors, first the hospital's Episcopalian chaplain, his curiosity doubtless aroused by the fact that I had jotted "Anglican" as my religion on my forms. He left me several pamphlets, but had no suggestion for the pain. A well-dressed older man appeared a little later, introducing himself as a former patient who had been operated on several years before and was now—as he was sure I would be—"clean as a whistle." He had the eyes of a door-to-door salesman, and I wondered what, exactly, he was selling. He was, it turned out, distributing applications to join the Friends of Patrick Walsh, the organization devoted to fund-raising for further research into prostate cancer at Johns Hopkins. He showed me a helpful chart illustrating exactly what the tax savings would be if I chose to donate $50,000, or $100,000, or $1 million, spread out over so many years. I told him that I would think it over, but I could tell he wasn't satisfied. He wanted a pledge, or at least a signature, but I pleaded fatigue until I finally succeeded in driving him away, at least for the moment. I was sure he would be back.

The most exciting part of the morning was when I was helped out of bed into my dressing gown and slippers and sent off to plod back and forth down the corridor, pushing my IV stand in front of me, arm-in-arm with a nurse. Walking was hard work—each shuffling step seemed to require superhuman strength; still, it felt good to be on my feet again. I passed Ned, in a checked dressing gown, shuffling crablike in the opposite direction. He looked about twenty years older than he had the last time I saw him, and I suppose the same was true of me. I looked in on Bob, who was watching television, red-faced and cheerful, a living testimonial to morphine.

By the time I got back to my freshly made bed and was helped into it, I was exhausted. I could not have walked for more than ten minutes at a snail's pace, but I felt as if I had run a marathon. Worse still, the pain was as bad as ever. By the time Margaret arrived, to find me picking away at my lunch, I was beginning to feel desperate. Pushing the pain button had no effect whatsoever, and nobody seemed to believe me. The Pain Team had not appeared, despite my many requests to the day nurses. Margaret went off to the nurses' station to put out an SOS for them, to no avail.

It was not until late in the afternoon that they showed up, cheerful as only specialists can be. One look was enough to tell them what the problem was. The computer that metered my dosage was not programmed correctly. That was why, when I pushed my pain button, nothing happened. The system had been fine when they left yesterday, they said. The nurses must have fiddled around with the buttons. It happened all the time.

I was in no mood for turf warfare—I already knew what the nurses, on their side, thought of the Pain Team. Just get it set up right, I asked. The Pain Team leader shrugged. Not a problem, he said. A child could do it. It was dead simple, if only the nurses would leave it be. . . .

He fiddled with the box; I pushed the button, and felt, at last, almost instantaneous relief.

I felt somehow cheated. Bob, in the room down the corridor, had been floating happily on a sea of morphine since his surgery. Ned's pain machine had worked like a charm. I had been connected to mine for twenty-four hours without deriving much benefit from it. I wanted the Valium I had been promised for my bladder cramps, but this, too, was a problem. Instructions had been left, but they had not been issued, and only a doctor could do it. Repeated requests produced nothing, except increasing ill will, which I was anxious to avoid. Margaret, after all, could go back to her hotel. I was stuck here, at the mercy of the staff. Finally Margaret discovered two young interns lounging in their green scrub suits at the nurses' station, to whom she explained my need for Valium. They continued their conversation. It was—or seemed at the time to be—the last straw. She turned on them with the fury of a woman who is being ignored and screamed, "I want my husband's Valium! Now!"

I heard her, from my bed, and was not surprised that I got my Valium a few minutes later, only twenty-four hours more or less since I had been promised it. It worked, too. Very shortly, the bladder cramps stopped. That night I was actually able to eat a helping of meat loaf, with gravy and mashed potatoes. It wasn't bad meat loaf, either, as meat loaf goes. What goes in *has* to go out, I prayed.

—⁓—

KEN ARETSKY TURNED out to be a better judge of the situation than anybody else. He had told me that the second night was the worst, that he had reached his personal nadir early on the third morning after surgery, and he was absolutely right.

Partly, I think, it was a question of the crisis wearing off. Obviously, I was in no danger. Clearly, my cancer had been dealt with. I was therefore no longer protected by adrenaline, or a sense of drama—my body was gradually waking up to the enormous trauma that had been inflicted on it. At the same time, a new and much harder pain had emerged now that I was eating again: gas, which I had no way of passing yet, swelled and pressed against my sutures and stitches, an immovable block of agony that left me doubled up, clutching my stomach, tears in my eyes. It had been explained to me that part of the reason for getting the patient up on his feet is that walking helps to get the gas moving, but despite walking, mineral oil, and milk of magnesia, mine wasn't going anywhere, and until it did, it was going to hurt like hell.

That second night seemed endlessly long and lonely. I missed David, now off duty, and his personal touch. I lay rigid, unwilling to move, clutching the frame of the bed until my knuckles ached, staring out into the corridor, listening to the sharp ping of warning bells and buzzers, waiting for dawn.

At best, sleep is hard in hospitals. Bells ring, people moan and groan, and just as one *is* about to doze off somebody is sure to arrive to take one's temperature and blood pressure, or replace the IV bag, or empty the drains and catheter bag. Everybody knows this about hospitals, and by and large it's true. What people mostly *don't* comment on is that most of the nurses do their best to make the patient comfortable.

All things considered, if there's one thing about the modern hospital that *does* work—apart from the technology itself—it's the nurses. Harassed, brutally overworked, for the most part poorly paid, they were unfailingly cheerful and helpful. Whenever they saw me walking up and down the corridor, pushing my IV before me, they would call out cheerfully, "Head up!"; for slouching, head down, did no good—you had to walk at as brisk a pace as you could manage, head held high, to give the digestive tract a chance to work. From time to time one of them would place a stethoscope against my stomach and listen hopefully for bowel sounds. The more noise from the bowels, the better the prognosis for a bowel movement, or the movement of something, *anything*. So far, there was only silence.

—m—

THE EARLY HOURS of the morning seem to drag on forever in a hospital. You lie there in the dim light from the corridor, alone with your own fears and discomfort and pointless second thoughts. (Why did this happen to me? Why did I decide on surgery? What did I do to deserve this?)

Hours pass slowly, wakefully, then it's time for the nurses on the night shift to get the patients ready for the day shift, and the tempo picks up. The patients are washed, given a toothbrush and a glass to rinse out with, handed their electric razor. IV bags are changed, catheter bags and drains emptied. Sleep is now out of the question, as are glum thoughts. Everybody is busy tidying, completing charts, getting the patients to sit up with as much animation as they can manage. It's cleanup time.

Some things are easier to clean than others. The Foley catheter was a bitch—by no means maintenance-free. Obviously, the bag had to be emptied from time to time, but the catheter tube also had to be cleaned at frequent intervals, sterilized with alcohol pads and coated with Neomycin ointment. The penis and the first couple of inches of the tube as it emerged from the urethra then had to be wrapped with a surgical gauze pad, over which an absorbent pad was rolled, the whole thing then firmly held in place with surgical tape. I was urged to watch this procedure carefully, since I would soon be doing it myself—which at last made clear why I had been advised to lay in a quantity of these medical supplies for my return home.

I was dismayed by the fact that the catheter *leaked*. Some catheter tubes, it was explained to me, were a better fit in the urethra than others. Besides which, the bladder, particularly when it was in spasm, pushed harder than it needed to, thus forcing urine out at a faster rate than the catheter could cope with. The overflow came out the meatus in the form of a steady drip, and an occasional flood.

In my case, just as Dr. Walsh had warned, the situation would not be helped by the fact that my history of prostate enlargement had made my bladder stronger and more muscular than it now needed to be. Before, the bladder had been obliged to push hard to force urine down a narrowed urethra; now, there was nothing to block or impede the flow of urine, but the bladder had no way of knowing that. Its walls, the muscle thickened by years of exertion, were pushing as hard as ever.

Cleaning it did nothing to relieve the leakage, of course. That did not bother me too much so long as I was lying in bed, but when I stood up and walked I left a trail of bloody urine behind me on the floor. The nurses didn't seem to mind. This was a urology ward, after all, and bloody urine on the floor was par for the course. I, on the other hand, minded deeply. It offended the fastidious side of my nature, which I found hard to let go of. I felt somehow shamed, humiliated, soiled, no longer an adult in full control of my bodily functions—all the more so since neither Ned nor Bob seemed to be suffering from the same problem. I got the somewhat depressing impression that fastidiousness was going to be something of a losing battle over the next few weeks, or possibly longer. A distaste for intimate contact with one's own body wastes is normal, even healthy—we all had that dinned into us when we were toilet trained, so it's right down in the bedrock of the subconscious, written in stone—but it was beginning to occur to me that anyone undergoing a radical prostatectomy had better get over that as quickly as possible.

Whatever else was going to happen, I decided, I was going to be in closer contact with my own urine than had been the case since my infancy.

I didn't like the idea a bit.

—⁓—

BREAKFAST BROUGHT WITH it the only moment at which a decision was called for from me: my choice from the lunch and the supper menus. People make fun of hospital food, but as anybody who has experienced this kind of surgery can attest, the mere idea of being *able* to eat, of feeling interested enough in food to make a choice, represents a huge step back to normal.

As I munched my cornflakes slowly, I read the day's menu with loving attention. So the "garden salad bowl" would consist mostly of faded iceberg lettuce, with a plastic pouch of French's Italian dressing on the side, so what? I put a tick in that box, happy to be making a choice. So the beef stew would be lukewarm, and straight out of a can, who cared? Here at least was something that called for a decision, something *normal*—for what could be more normal than choosing from a menu? I might have no control over my bowels, which were still firmly stoppered, or over my urine, which leaked every time I stood up, but I could choose beef stew, and know that it would arrive on my tray, even if it was accompanied by limp, gray string beans and pasty mashed potatoes. I regarded the menus as a kind of link to life, and although I was not in the least hungry, I would happily have sent my compliments to the chef. Besides, for me, brought up on "nursery food," the hospital menu was like old times. Where else, these days, do you find Jell-O, rice pudding, and bananas on a menu?

That I was able to think about food—thinking about it was a lot easier than eating it still—was a good sign, proof, I thought, that I was firmly on Ken Aretsky's schedule, in which case the worst was behind me.

And so it proved. I still felt awful, but at some point during the course of the third day, I actually managed to get up, make my own way to the bathroom, and have a bowel movement, together with a release of gas that promised substantial relief for that pain, at least. This had been a point that Professor Martin celebrated in his book, and now I understood why—it's the first sign that *something* is recovering, the down payment, as it were, on one's ticket out of the hospital.

17

THE THIRD DAY WAS NOTABLE FOR A NEW DIFFERENCE OF OPINION with Dr. Walsh, this one brought about by a doctor friend from New York who, with her husband, had come down to Baltimore to visit me and take Margaret out to dinner. Our friend had heard from Margaret about my problems with pain management, and felt strongly that there was no reason for me to have been suffering. She had tried to reach Dr. Walsh in the morning to clarify what my pain medication was supposed to be, but they had failed to make contact. She was therefore unaware that the problem had been solved, and since I was sleeping, I wasn't able to tell her.

Since his encounter with Margaret, Dr. Walsh did not, I felt sure, look upon his visit to me as the happiest moment of his rounds. It was therefore, perhaps, unfortunate that when Dr. Walsh made his rounds that evening, shortly after I woke up, my friend and her husband were in my room, about to take Margaret out to yet another meal of Maryland crab cakes. After a ritual handshake like that between two boxers in the ring, she waded in immediately. Now that he was here, she wanted to know the protocol for my pain medication. Dr. Walsh tried treating this lightly, but his face was stony. "You're a lucky man," he told me. "This is the first time I've ever seen a doctor make a house call all the way from New York." I smiled nervously, feeling something of a traitor.

She, however, was not to be fobbed off with a joke. She wanted to know what the protocol was for my pain medication, she explained, because judging from what she had heard she did not think it had been followed. She wondered, in fact, if the Pain Management Unit had been following Dr. Walsh's instructions.

The suggestion that he might not know what was going on in his own hospital brought an instant glow to Dr. Walsh's face, and the light of battle into his eyes. The two doctors confronted each other, Dr. Walsh having the advantage of height and home turf, my friend with a certain bulldog tenacity, coupled with sweet reason, that I had never seen her display before. Of course, since they were doctors, they were bound by the rules of their profession, which demand a display of politeness, however icy, before laypersons. Dr. Walsh emphasized politely that he was in charge and that my operation had been, as promised, a great success. It was important to keep in mind what really mattered. She pointed out that while all that was no doubt true, it still did not explain the failure of the pain management, and that this might be something Dr. Walsh should look into.

Dr. Walsh directed himself to me, with a certain steady indignation in his voice. Had I any reason to be dissatisfied? If I had any complaints, I should address them to *him,* not to another doctor. *Did* I have any complaints? Feeling like a complete coward now, I weakly conveyed my satisfaction. My friend waved me to silence. I was in no condition to speak for myself. No doubt the operation was a success, she had never questioned that, but there had been a problem with pain medication here, and it ought to be looked into.

That night the nurses positively tiptoed around my bed, as if I had committed some form of medical lèse-majesté. Some of the more outspoken ones even expressed a certain guarded admiration for my doctor friend, perhaps because in urology most of the nurses are still women (David was an exception), while most of the doctors are men. Hospitals are hierarchical to a degree almost unknown in ordinary life outside the military, and no doctor is in the habit of being questioned, let alone one as eminent and powerful as Patrick Walsh. Luckily for me, whatever blame was floating around over the incident was attributed to the Pain Team, who, since they were out of the direct doctor/nurse/patient loop and apparently spent their day wandering from ward to ward through the vast hospital, relentlessly pursued by beeped messages, could be blamed for anything that went wrong without their even knowing it.

—⚹—

THEY CERTAINLY DIDN'T bear a grudge, though from my point of view my next close encounter with them was something of a disappointment. They reappeared in my room the next morning with all their equipment, cheerful and smiling as ever, bearing the good news that since my pain medication was now working satisfactorily, it was time to remove it.

I protested feebly (Margaret's protests were considerably less feeble) but to no avail. After all, I argued, for more than twenty-four hours I had been deprived of pain relief. Surely I was entitled to an extra day, or even half a day? But no. The schedule must be adhered to rigidly, and by the schedule it was time to remove the epidural IV from my back, whether I felt pain or not.

I was so incensed at the unfairness of this that I failed even to notice the removal of the epidural, which I had feared almost as much as its insertion. It was simply plucked out, like a dart being pulled from a dartboard, and that was that.

The Pain Team left, taking with them my "pain box" and all the tubing that had attached me to it. I felt a curious combination of anger and relief—anger that the system was so inflexible, and at the irony of having the "pain box" removed as soon as it was working the way it was supposed to; relief that one more gadget tying me to the hospital was gone.

By the fourth day, I was beginning to be more conscious of my appearance—definitely a good sign. I had shaved myself from the start, but now I waited desperately for my morning sponge bath, and a change of gown, and hated putting on my bathrobe and slippers, both of which, inevitably, were stained with dried blood and urine.

Walking was still an effort, but I no longer returned to my bed trembling and out of breath after a few minutes, and I was able to get into bed myself, even managing somehow to swing my legs back up onto the bed. I could walk for half an hour or more without distress, although there was still a natural tendency to let my head droop, which Margaret and the nurses vigorously corrected. Head up, shoulders back, stomach in, they kept telling me, and while it was difficult to do, they were right.

I had grown used to the tight anti-embolism socks, and to the importance of keeping my legs raised on a pillow, and I could even make it to the bathroom by myself now, though with great difficulty, dragging my bag, my drains, and my tubes after me, and constantly getting them tangled up with the cords of the call button and the telephone. I worried, when I was seated in the dark and dismal little bathroom, whether I would be able to get back up again and into bed, and sometimes it was a struggle that left me close to tears from sheer frustration, but I cherished the minor victory of independence.

More than anything else, I wanted to go home—a good sign, I think. The only people, after all, who want to be in a hospital are those who are *really* sick—those too sick to be comfortable or to survive elsewhere. I was no longer in that category.

Dr. Walsh had indicated that I would be leaving "on schedule," in two days' time. If it was deemed necessary, I would be asked to stay an extra night in Baltimore, at the hotel, and come in for a checkup the next day, before returning home. This was the very last thing I wanted to do, of course. I wasn't sure just *how* I was going to get home, but once I was out of the hospital I didn't want to hang around Baltimore in a hotel room, in some sort of overnight limbo.

As I shuffled up and down the corridor, still tangled up in my plastic tubes, I tried to imagine myself waiting for an airplane to arrive at the Pittsburgh airport (probably hours late), or sitting in an airplane for hours while it circled La Guardia in bad weather. Admittedly, I would be moved around the airport in a wheelchair by a porter, but I still couldn't imagine how I was going to make it. When it came to travel, Dr. Walsh sent out conflicting signals. I had thought it might be a good idea to avoid the problems of air travel altogether by hiring a car and driver to take me home, door to door. That, however, turned out to be a nonstarter. Sitting for long periods was the one thing I shouldn't be doing any more than was absolutely necessary, in order to prevent embolism. Why couldn't I simply lie down across the backseat, with my legs propped up? I asked. But the answer to that was that Dr. Walsh didn't want me to be bumped around. I could understand *that* all right—I didn't want to be bumped around myself—but would it be any worse than taking a taxi from Johns Hopkins to the Baltimore airport, being wheeled to the plane, possibly subjected to a bumpy flight (*two* bumpy flights, actually), then driven from La Guardia home, a two-hour drive over some of the more deeply potholed roads of the entire northeastern United States?

As the hours passed I became more and more obsessed with the problem. A part of me felt that if I could just get moving, I could grit my teeth and keep moving somehow until I was home; another part of me couldn't imagine even taking the first step. Margaret, who was spending her days helping me walk up and down the hospital corridors, was even more concerned about my ability to travel than I was. In the end it was she who made a call to Richard and Roxanne Bacon, back home, to talk about it, and Richard who mentioned that he had a niece who was a nurse on a medevac plane. The moment I heard about this, my anxiety lifted. The medevac people, it turned out, would arrange the whole trip. An ambulance would pick us up at Johns Hopkins and take us to the Baltimore airport; a small plane, equipped with a stretcher, and with a fully qualified nurse on board, would fly us to the small airport nearest our house; and another ambulance would deliver me home, perhaps a twenty-minute drive. For the first time I had a sense of being in control, of *making arrangements.* I was on the phone, reading off my credit card number, setting up a schedule, sounding, I have no doubt, like a hysteric—all the more so since my voice had been reduced to a hoarse, breathless wheeze. (Somewhere along the way, I had simply lost the ability to speak normally. Everybody assured me that it would return, but in the meantime anybody listening to me trying to speak above a whisper would have thought that my problem had been lung cancer, not prostate cancer.)

Up to that point, I had been afraid of what it would be like to *leave* the hospital; now I was only afraid that the weather would delay our departure, or that Dr. Walsh would decree that I had to stay an extra day.

—∿—

BUT DR. WALSH did no such thing—was perhaps happy, it occurred to me later, to see Margaret and me go. We went through the standard departure checklist, step by step, the first being the hardest, for before anything else could happen, my drains and my staples had to be removed. My IV had already been removed, at last, and at the appointed hour an intern arrived, looking far too young for my liking. (Has he done this before? How often? Does he know what he's doing?) I asked if it was going to hurt. No, he said, he didn't think taking the staples out would hurt at all. Some people didn't like it when the drains came out, but it was all over in a second.

I remembered that in Professor Martin's book, *My Prostate and Me,* one of his friends had described this as "the most excruciatingly unpleasant" moment of his hospital stay, remarking that it had felt as if his "intestines were being pulled out," while a nurse said that most men compared it to "sticking their finger in a light socket." That didn't sound good.

The intern examined my incision, which so far I had resisted looking at myself, but which I could now see in the form of a row of shiny metal staples from my navel to my penis, holding together a cut as straight as an autobahn. I had expected to be nauseated by the sight of my own flesh cut like a side of beef. To my surprise, however, I felt nothing much, except that the sheer size of the incision made it clear just how "major" this kind of surgery was. The young man admired it with starry eyes. "Pat Walsh," he said, shaking his head in awe. "*Nice* work!"

He carefully cut each staple, starting from the top, deftly removing both bits and dropping them into a tray with a flourish and a sharp *ping*. As he removed each staple, he covered the tiny holes with a small Band-Aid. These, he assured me, would not come off for some time, but when they did, I was to let them go.

When he had finished, he told me to shut my eyes. I did, and felt a sudden, strange pull deep inside me, not exactly painful, but somehow as if a tree were being uprooted in my abdomen. Things were being pulled and twisted and moved in there that ought to have been left in peace—that was the closest I could come to describing the sensation, which, while it was nothing like as bad as I had feared, was on the other hand not anything I would ever want to experience again. "That's it," the intern said cheerfully. "All done."

Without the drains, I felt a good deal freer. Above all, it felt good not to see them all the time, the bloody liquid that filled them at regular intervals an all-too-vivid reminder of what the surgery was really about.

For the first time I really believed that I was going home.

18

THE EVENING OF MY LAST FULL DAY IN THE HOSPITAL I RECEIVED good news. I could go *directly* home—I would not have to spend an extra night in Baltimore, after all. On the other hand, the weather report for the next day was terrible—sleet, snow, fog, freezing rain. Alarmed, I called the medevac people. Not to worry, they said. They would have a plane in Baltimore by late afternoon, whatever the weather was like. I breathed a sigh of relief.

The next morning, we received our final instructions. My urologist at home would remove the catheter in three weeks' time. (How would *that* feel? I wondered.) If the catheter should come loose, I was to go to the emergency room of the nearest hospital immediately, so that it could be reinserted. To make sure it *didn't* come loose, I should renew the tape that held the tube to my thigh at frequent intervals. In the event of a sudden fever, I was to call a doctor right away. Margaret and I were shown how to put on the anti-embolism stockings—the chief thing to remember was to put plenty of baby powder on the legs before trying to pull them on, since they were a very tight fit—and were presented with three pairs. I was shown how to empty the urine bag and how to replace the big bag with the smaller, flask-shaped leg bag, for walking around or going to the movies. (Going to the *movies*? Who had even *imagined* going to the movies again like a normal human being?) I was also shown how to wash and clean the catheter bags, and was given a supply, a kind of starter kit, of alcohol pads, Neomycin, surgical tape and pad, and antibiotics to prevent infection. I was firmly warned that I must continue to take milk of magnesia and mineral oil every night because any straining to produce a bowel movement could rupture the delicate stitches inside me—this was a serious business, it was emphasized, and I took it as such. With that, I was helped into my street clothes, while the bed in my room was stripped, to be made ready for another patient that evening.

We were not out of the woods yet. As if this were some kind of black comedy, we simply couldn't get out of Johns Hopkins now that we were ready to leave it. The ambulance had gone to Margaret's hotel, and could not be traced. I paced clumsily up and down the hall, dragging my urine bag behind me, trying to make contact with somebody, *anybody,* on my cellular telephone, while the hours crept past. It was an odd feeling. Ned and Gladys, Bob and Gail, had all said their good-byes and gone, a new shift of nurses had appeared. I was no longer a part of this little community, neither a patient now nor a visitor; I was suddenly invisible. The nurses were friendly enough, but I was no longer their problem.

At last, the ambulance turned up. I was put in a wheelchair, my bag placed in my lap, and we set off on a marathon journey through Johns Hopkins to the main entrance. It was late now, and dark. I had hoped to fly in the daylight—our local airport is not exactly a cow patch, but it isn't La Guardia, either, and approaching it on a sleeting, icy night wasn't an idea I would normally embrace, except that by now I no longer cared.

Once we had found the ambulance, I was lifted into it and strapped onto a stretcher, and we set off through the rain toward the airport. To my distress, the driver promptly got lost. We rushed down deserted streets, stopped, backed up, rushed in the other direction, all to no avail. From time to time we actually entered the airport only to find that we were in the international cargo area or some other dark or brightly floodlit dead end. Once, we actually crossed a runway, and I had visions of a head-on crash with a Boeing 737. The driver put on his flashing lights, then put on his siren, but the faster we went, the more hopelessly lost we became.

I was beginning to suffer from anxiety. Would the plane wait for us? Would I have to go back to the hospital or the hotel, and start out all over again in the morning? Would I ever get home? The nurse—a huge and gentle black man—held my hand and calmed me by taking my blood pressure every few minutes as we careened like bank robbers around Baltimore's airport. Finally, we arrived at the private aviation area and pulled up before a small aircraft with a scream of brakes.

I glanced out the window. A freezing rain was falling. Within minutes, I was tucked inside a blanket in the small airplane, and we were airborne, bumping and thrashing through the turbulent skies—just the thing Pat Walsh had forbidden, I reflected. The flight nurse took my blood pressure at regular intervals, too, a strangely comforting feeling, perhaps because it gives one the sense that one is being *cared* for, monitored, even if it's unnecessary.

By twisting my head, I could see Margaret and the pilot sitting together up front, while rain and sleet beat against the windscreen. "Pretty marginal down there," the pilot shouted cheerfully.

"I don't care," I said. "I just want to sleep in my own bed tonight."

"Amen to *that*," the pilot said, and shortly afterward we swooped through the clouds and fog and landed with a splash on the flooded runway of our local airport, sending up sheets of water as if we were in a seaplane.

An ambulance waited—local boys, this time, who knew the way to our house. I saw Richard Bacon, who had come to meet us, and gave him a weak wave of the hand. The next thing I remember, the two ambulance men were carrying me up the stairs in a fireman's carry and depositing me in my own bed.

I was home.

I didn't know it, but the hard part was about to begin.

PART THREE

RECUPERATION

19

SO LONG AS YOU'RE IN THE HOSPITAL, YOUR RECUPERATION IS IN other people's hands. Once you're home, it's your own problem.

Note that I use the word *recuperation*—that is to say, getting over the surgery and back to life and work. *Recovery* is a different (and more long-term) matter, as much in the mind as in the body, and will be dealt with later.

Some hint of what was in store during the recuperative phase was that the home care nurse had been waiting for us at the house, just to make sure that I was okay. Service, I thought, over and above the call of duty, congratulating myself on having thought something out in advance.

All the doctors I had talked to before the operation had pooh-poohed my questions about home nursing care. I wouldn't need a nurse, there wasn't anything Margaret and I couldn't handle by ourselves, it was a waste of money and of valuable nursing time, etc. Quite apart from my skepticism about all this—do doctors have any understanding of how their patients actually live, in the real world?—

I could not help noticing that my insurance company was perfectly willing to pay for two months of regular visits to my home by a nurse, as well as two months of home care by a nurse's aide. Considering that the same insurance company wanted me out of the hospital after a maximum of four days, which had outraged Dr. Walsh, who wrote to them indignantly to say that he considered five days the absolute minimum, it seemed to me a good bet that the nursing care was probably going to be necessary. After all, insurance companies these days don't go in for the superfluous or the frivolous.

Laura Mansfield, the nurse, was a smart, personable, cheerful, and competent young woman with a brisk sense of humor—she exuded a kind of "tough love" attitude (as opposed to the "mommy" approach), which was exactly what I needed. She took my blood pressure (for the umpteenth time that day) and my temperature, changed my dressings, then explained that she would be visiting me every morning to take my vital signs and report any problems to my doctor. If I had an emergency, I was to call her service night or day, and they would beep her. When she came back the next morning, she would also brief my nurse's aide. The nurse's aide would be with me from eight in the morning until early afternoon, and would help me bathe, dress, care for my catheter, and exercise. She would also shop for me, when necessary, and prepare light meals, though on that score, I would do well not to have exaggerated expectations. Would I be needing the nurse's aide to clip my toenails? If so, I should tell the nurse's aide.

I said I could probably handle that myself, feeling a little like somebody who was living under false pretenses. I wasn't *that* sick, after all—although, now that I gave the matter some thought, how *was* I going to clip my toenails when the time came? I could not bend over, not with an abdominal incision nearly nine inches long. What other small, ordinary human needs and activities that I had not even considered would I also be unable to do? Washing my hair leapt to mind. Pulling my trousers on over my wraps, dressings, and catheter tube? I *knew* that was going to be a tough one.

Laura examined the changes Richard Bacon and our friend Dot Burnett had made in the house—the bathroom with the bathtub seat, the handrails and the hand shower, the rubber-backed mats covering the carpets everywhere I might walk—and gave her approval. Lots of people didn't think of these things beforehand, she said, then when they returned home from the hospital it was too late. Had I had anything to drink? she asked.

I shook my head. I had deliberately avoided taking a lot of fluid— the more you drink, the more you pee, and I didn't want to add any complications to my trip. Besides, I hadn't been thirsty.

Laura was shocked. Hadn't anybody told me that my intake of fluid had to be kept as high as possible? Five or six thousand milliliters a day (the equivalent of a dozen glasses), *at least,* and without fail, she added sternly. Also, I was to keep a record of exactly how many ounces of liquid I took in and how much liquid had accumulated in the catheter bag before I emptied it. Output was as important as input. I was not to cheat. She would be checking the numbers every day.

Even in my exhausted and woozy state, I found this interesting. Apart from a generalized recommendation to drink plenty of fluids, nobody at Johns Hopkins had suggested that my liquid intake and urine output had to be monitored carefully, or even mattered that much. I had been turned loose with a single sheet of instructions, in the form of a printed letter from Dr. Walsh which I now dug out of my briefcase. It warned against lifting anything heavier than ten pounds for six weeks after surgery (this might lead to a hernia in the incision, or worse yet, disrupt the anastomosis—the healing that was taking place between the stump of the urethra and the bladder, which had been sewn together around the neck of the catheter) and emphasized the danger of embolism during the first four to six weeks after surgery. I was not to drive a car until eight weeks after surgery.

The third paragraph had caught my attention, since it contained the underlined sentence "Do not become discouraged!" This paragraph dealt with incontinence, and remarked that "problems with urinary control are common once the catheter is removed." Control, Dr. Walsh promised, would return in three distinct phases. First I would be dry when I was lying down at night; then I'd stay dry even when I was walking around; the final phase would be when I remained dry when rising from the seated position. To speed up the return of continence, I should practice shutting off and restarting the flow of urine while standing, contracting the buttocks muscles tightly. I should do this *only* while urinating, so as not to tire the sphincter muscles. I was absolutely *not* to do these exercises at any other time.

Dr. Walsh went into some detail in his letter about what to wear after the catheter had been removed. He recommended Depends, or a Confidence brief, both of which I had already stocked up on, but warned that under no circumstances should I wear an incontinence device, a condom catheter (a *what*?), or a clamp (a *clamp*?). I should avoid drinking "excessive amounts of fluids," he advised, and limit my intake of alcohol and caffeine.

Erections, Dr. Walsh promised, on a more cheerful note, would return gradually. I was to be "patient." Some men did not recover potency until two years after surgery. I would find that "visual and psychogenic stimuli" would be less effective and "tactile sensation will be more effective"—food for thought!—which I took to mean that pornography and sexually arousing situations would be less effective in producing an erection than direct physical touch and stimulation of the penis. That didn't sound too bad.

There was more—though in my present state it was only of remote interest. There would be no emission during orgasm—that, I already knew—and many men found that they lost their erections when they attempted orgasm, a problem which could be solved by using Coban tape (which "doesn't stick to the hair") in strips half an inch wide to make a tourniquet at the base of the penis. Coban tape was widely available at drugstores and pharmacies, which suggested to me that its use was not confined to those who had had a radical prostatectomy.

Dr. Walsh gave the patient his telephone numbers—including his home phone in case of problems on the weekends, which impressed me. I had already been booked to have my first telephone conversation with him two months after the operation, and further regular conversations would be arranged at four-month intervals for the first year following surgery, then at six-month or yearly intervals. In closing, he wished me good luck, and added "You have had a good operation and you will do well."

I found it interesting that Dr. Walsh advised *against* excessive fluid intake in his instructions, and I said so to Laura. She took the letter and read it. She handed it back scornfully. "Doctors!" she said. "What do they know?"

They knew how to perform an operation, sure, she went on, but after that, forget it. Fluid intake was *vital,* and that was that. She also took issue with Dr. Walsh about the exercises. The more I exercised the sphincter muscles, once the catheter had been removed, the quicker continence would return. She gave me a pamphlet (written by a nurse, of course) describing "Kegel exercises," named after Dr. Walter Kegel. Read it carefully, she said. Recuperation wasn't going to happen all by itself, and wouldn't come easy.

MARGARET HAD HELPED me undress, washed me, and put me to bed—no small task, as it turned out. I had to be firmly positioned on a rubber, leakproof mat, with another one on top of me, to prevent wetting either the sheet below me or the one above; my catheter bag had to be placed just so on the floor, so that nobody would step on it and I wouldn't trip on it; my legs, sprinkled with baby powder and firmly encased in anti-embolism socks, had to be raised on two hard pillows. I had developed the habit—an obsession—of covering myself with my dressing gown, as if I were wrapped in a cocoon, which for some reason, perhaps vaguely derived from the nursery, I found comforting. By the time I was ready for sleep, movement of any kind was by no means easy—I was firmly wedged into position. And yet I would have to move if I started to leak urine too badly, or if my catheter bag filled up. The latter had not yet happened, but would be signaled by the fact that urine would start backing up in my bladder once the bag was full, at which point, as Laura had put it, I would "know about it in a hurry." I didn't like the sound of that, but it turned out to be on the money.

I slept uneasily, while Margaret, usually a poor sleeper, lay beside me on the unprotected side of our bed, unconscious from sheer exhaustion and stress. It was our first night together since the one before the operation, and I couldn't help reflecting on the change in my situation. *Then*, we had slept in each other's arms after making love. *Now*, we were on separate sides of the bed, with me stretched out uneasily on and under layers of leakproof mats, my catheter tube connecting me to a large plastic urine bag on the floor beside my slippers. It was not the way I had envisioned life during the celebration of my sixtieth birthday, only a little more than a year before.

I had prepared myself for a lot, but what I was *not* prepared for, now that I was home again, was the way in which the least interesting and most normal of everyday bodily functions had taken over my life, almost to the exclusion of everything else. The hospital had given me a taste of it, but then you *expect* that in a hospital, it's part of the experience—tubes, drains, catheters, bedpans, and urinals are par for the course.

At home, it's different. At home, you can compare what life was like *before* with what it's like *now*. Urine, I could see, was now my major concern, the element around which much of my life was going to revolve—for how long? The floors were covered with mats, partly to make sure I didn't slip, to be sure, but also to protect the carpets in case I dripped urine. The leakproof mattress cover on the bed, and the rubber-backed pad above and below me, were to keep the bed dry in case of "an accident" or "a problem." There was a notepad in the bathroom so that I could write down exactly how much urine the catheter bag contained each time I emptied it. Until the catheter was removed it was going to be the most familiar and intimate presence in my life.

Nobody with a catheter is really incontinent—the catheter drains the bladder constantly, without any intervention or interruption. Still, the full meaning of the word *incontinence* hadn't quite dawned on me until now—oh, I knew what it *meant,* all right, but *experiencing* it was quite a different matter, and the catheter gave me a foretaste of just what it would be like, not so much in the physical sense as the mental. It meant that there wasn't a moment, day or night, that you weren't *conscious* of your urine, weren't thinking about it, weren't concerned that you were leaking it, or dripping it, or that other people could smell it on you, no matter how much you washed, and scrubbed the catheter tube with alcohol pads, and sprayed Lysol everywhere around you. . . . From being Topic Z, way down at the bottom of anybody's list of daily concerns, it had leapt right up there to Topic B or C, if you took cancer as A, by a long shot, and included impotence on the list.

Apart from cancer itself, it had been impotence that terrified me most before the operation, but the reality was that incontinence was in some ways worse—in any case, I wondered, what good would potency be if you were still incontinent? Who would want to have sex with a man who couldn't control his bladder—who might leak urine at any moment? It would be hard to imagine anything more anaphrodisiac than *that.* . . .

Of course, I told myself, there are worse things, *much* worse. The cancer might have spread to the lymph nodes or, God forbid, to the bones, and it still might; for despite Dr. Walsh's optimism, I had read the statistics and knew there were no guarantees. When prostate cancer reaches the bones, death comes in its grimmest form, the patient often suffering fractures merely from being gently moved in bed, uncontrollable pain spreading through his body, total paralysis of life functions. . . . You have to look on the bright side, I reminded myself, avoid self-pity, remind yourself that getting rid of the cancer is objective number one, dwarfing every other problem.

But in the middle of the night, it's hard to look on the bright side of *anything.* I told myself again that nobody had given me any guarantees; I had gone into this with my eyes open, knowing what the consequences of the surgery might be, had actually signed off on them on the dotted line just before the anesthesiologists had arrived to take me into the operating room. Incontinence was part of the package, and most men suffered from it to one degree or another after surgery, ditto impotence. Mostly you got over them, more or less.

"Do not become discouraged!" Dr. Walsh had written in his farewell letter to patients leaving for home, and I was determined *not* to become discouraged. One had to be *patient*, I understood that. Continence, I told myself, would return slowly, but surely; potency, perhaps a good deal slower and less surely, would follow—except in a small percentage of cases. . . . Well, luck, as always, would play a role. I remembered Professor Martin's book. *He* had experienced almost no incontinence; *his* catheter hadn't leaked a bit; *he* had had an erection while he was still in the hospital, with the catheter still in him! Throughout most of life, I thought, my luck had been pretty good—certainly when it came to health. There was no reason to suppose that I wouldn't be one of the lucky ones who regained continence almost as soon as the catheter was out, and whose potency returned ahead of schedule.

I dozed off, sweaty and uncomfortable under all my layers of coverings, and dreamed, of all things, that I was standing in front of a urinal in the men's room of a restaurant, desperate to pee, but unable to, while all around me people—men, some of them vaguely familiar; *women,* too—were gathered around me making suggestions about how to get the flow started. Somebody turned on all the taps, in the hope that the sound of running water would do the trick, somebody else flushed the toilets, but nothing happened. I could feel the urine backing up in me, as if my bladder were full to bursting, *as if it were about to explode!*

I woke with a start, and realized that the physical discomfort wasn't just a dream, it was painfully real. I reached down and felt the catheter bag on the floor. It was full, bulging at the seams with warm urine. Just as the nurse had warned, when it was full, you *knew* it.

Inspired by a desire to be self-sufficient, I pulled apart my bed-clothes, swung my legs over the side, and rose to my feet shakily. The Depends disposable pads were soaked. I gathered them up, put my robe over my shoulders, picked up my catheter bag, startled by how heavy it was, and stumbled into my bathroom. The catheter bag had what looked like a small spigot on the bottom. I wrote down how many milliliters of urine it contained, held it up over the toilet, turned the spigot, and emptied it. The swollen sensation in my bladder ebbed instantly. So far, so good.

I looked down. The dressings around the catheter, where it left the urethra, were soaked. They would have to be changed. I pulled the tape apart, removed the wet pad and the surgical dressing from the catheter tube, cleaned the tube with alcohol, slathered Neomycin on, replaced the dressings, and bound them up with enough surgical tape to make Johnson & Johnson stock rise a point. I then realized that I was standing in a pool of fresh urine. I had forgotten to close the spigot on the catheter bag.

By now I was alternating between angry cursing at my own stupidity and a rising inner pitch of anxiety that made my hands tremble. *Was this what I had come to? Was this what it was going to be like? And for how long? How could this be happening to me?*

I did not want to wake Margaret, who desperately needed (and deserved) her sleep. I sat down on the toilet, wiped the floor clean with paper towels, did my best to put everything away, then washed my hands (again) with antiseptic soap. I stumbled wearily back to bed, lay down on my pad, put two fresh Depends disposable pads above me, covering the dressing, placed another rubber-backed incontinence pad over *them,* then tucked my bathrobe up around my ears and tried to get back to sleep again.

My last thought before I finally fell asleep was that nobody had warned me about any of this. Professor Martin had not written about it in his book, nor had Dr. Rous in his, and Dr. Walsh had not mentioned it in his parting note. Clearly, there was going to be a lot more to recuperating than simply waiting for the body to return to normal, if it was, in fact, ever going to do that. And what would "normal" be? Would I regain 100 percent continence? 75 percent? Even if everything worked out as well as possible, I would still be a very *different* person, physically, from the one I had been, and perhaps emotionally as well. . . .

It occurred to me for the first time that perhaps the period *before* the surgery might be less difficult than the period *after* it. When the problem is *cancer*—and the surgery that you hope will get rid of it— there's a certain drama, a rush of adrenaline and excitement, however unwelcome, built into the situation. A crisis provides energy, places the cancer patient firmly at the center of other people's attention, has a rhythm to it: Act 1—diagnosis. Act 2—treatment. Act 3 (you hope)—cure: the crisis is over. Recuperation, on the other hand, lacks all that—it is an inherently untidy and undramatic process, with no timetable or rhythm to it at all. Who knows how long it will go on? Who can define the point at which it ends? Who can say when the patient has successfully recuperated—or if he really *has* recuperated, or has simply decided that that's it, enough, it's as good as it's going to get? There is a gray area between successful recuperation and the weary acceptance of one's new limits, and nobody but the patient himself can know how much baggage he has thrown overboard on the voyage before he finally reaches port.

Three weeks until the catheter is removed, I told myself.

I wondered how I was going to endure them.

The dressings were getting wet again—already. I had presumably taped them too loosely. The hell with it, I decided, and went back to sleep. The nurse's aide could take care of it in the morning, whoever she was.

———⁓———

BUT WHEN THE nurse's aide arrived, promptly at eight o'clock, it was in the person of Emory Smith, a chunky, cheerful, bespectacled young man in whites with the shoe-brush haircut of a military man. As it turned out, a military man was exactly what Emory was. He was a former U.S. Army medical corpsman who had served as a lieutenant in Gulf War combat. Emory and I quickly exchanged service careers, and settled almost immediately into a relationship which caused one observer to refer to us as "the Odd Couple."

Quite apart from the fact that men who have served in the military form a kind of international Freemasonry, Emory was a breath of fresh air. He might not be a doctor, but he knew all about wounds, incisions, and, particularly, catheters—it's hard to report sick with *anything* in the United States Armed Forces without being catheterized, if only because it keeps the patient quiet and establishes the authority of the nursing staff. More important, unlike doctors, Emory was willing, even *eager*, to talk. From him I got (at last) a sensible, practical picture of what progress I was likely to make and how long it would take, as well as a sense of how other prostate cancer patients he had looked after did and what *their* problems were.

It didn't hurt, either, that Emory, a natural storyteller, had looked after scores of people with problems far worse than my own, from young soldiers with AIDS to patients with Lou Gehrig's disease (ALS), to quadriplegics, to people in coma. Without ever coming right out and saying so, he deftly put my own fears and difficulties in perspective. I was going to get better—maybe not 100 percent better, but 50 or 60 percent. His previous patient, for example, who had ALS, could no longer feed himself, or swallow anything except special food that required no chewing, and would soon be unable to hold his head upright. Try living with *that*.

Emory seemed to get more than his share of the hard cases—in addition to which, he worked evenings and nights at a Catholic institution for mentally handicapped and violent children, from which he brought every morning a rich crop of horror stories. No kid was too autistic or violent, no patient too far gone, to defeat Emory's optimism, resourcefulness, and unshockability.

He took charge immediately. I hadn't given any thought to what my routine would be, so I fell into his, from day one. He got me out of bed, watched while I brushed my teeth and shaved, seated me in the bathtub while I used the hand shower, helped me dry myself off, and cast a soldierly eye on the way I took care of my catheter until I had it down to a routine. He helped me dress, solving the problem of getting the warm-up pants Margaret had bought me over the catheter tube, briskly powdering my legs so that he could pull on a clean pair of anti-embolism stockings, wrapping me up in a sweater, a parka, a watch cap, gloves—for, from the very beginning, I was determined to walk every morning whatever the weather, which in upstate New York in December is unlikely to be balmy. I cannot say that Emory approached this with enthusiasm—he was an armchair athlete—but he was not a soldier for nothing: putting one foot in front of the other was something he understood.

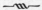

EVERYBODY EXCEPT MARGARET (who knew me—and herself—better) had urged me to go to Florida to recuperate. Sit by the pool, they said, bask in the sun, swim in lukewarm water, go for walks under the swaying palm trees, and I would mend easily, naturally, above all *comfortably.* I had resisted the whole idea—I wanted to be *home,* not in a hotel or a rented house; I wanted to get back to my normal routine, to my work, as soon as possible. I felt strongly that recuperation would come more quickly that way, that most of all I needed to regain control of *something* in my life, and that perhaps the only two areas in which I could hope to regain that control were exercise and work. Going to Florida was going in the wrong direction, or rather, going too far in the right direction: it was New York City I wanted to get back to, and my work.

So, from the very first morning, under a cold, gray sky, Emory, Margaret, and I, the three of us muffled to the gills against the cold, set off down the road outside our house, each of them holding on to an arm, as I shuffled breathlessly forward, trying to stand as upright as I could, holding my urine bag in a makeshift sling, determined to get to the end of our fenceline, perhaps a quarter of a mile away. I believed absolutely, without question, without doubt (and still believe), that that walk, lengthened every day, taken every morning even when the temperature plummeted and the windchill factor descended past the frostbite level, was what ultimately saved me from despair, fueled my recovery, brought me back at last from illness. One morning it was so cold that the urine in my bag froze solid—it made no difference; we went on. My morning walk was more than an obsession, it was a lifeline, and I grasped it with a desperation which only Margaret truly understood.

Mind, I do not say that you can make tissue heal any faster than it's going to, or will the bladder to accept the catheter, but you *can* walk, and each step takes you in the right direction. This was what I could do to contribute to my recuperation, physical and spiritual, and I was going to do it come hell or high water.

The urine bag was a contentious issue. Dr. Walsh recommended the use of the leg bag, a smaller, pouch-shaped, soft plastic container about the size of a paperback book that straps to the leg below the knee, for walking. The only trouble was—a hint, had I known it, of problems to come—that for some reason the urine backed up and leaked out of the catheter, soaking me, when I tried it. Emory and I rigged up a makeshift handle from strips of Velcro and I carried the big bag with me instead, like one of those string shopping bags elderly Frenchmen take to the market in the morning to hold their loaf of bread and bottle of wine.

Elderly, of course, was the operative word. I *felt* old, as if I had made a sudden leap into old age. I told myself that I would not have to imagine the problems of old age, that there would be no surprises when I got there—I was getting an early taste, from the slow, stumbling gait to the urinary problems. My voice was still low, cracked, a hoarse whisper. Why? Nobody knew. When would it get stronger? Nobody could say—and I got out of breath just walking upstairs, or getting up at night to empty my urine bag, and when I write "out of breath," I *mean* it: gasping as if I had just run a mile uphill.

I *looked* old, too—or a lot older, anyway. When I looked in the mirror, I saw a stranger, an old man from my posture to the dark bags under my eyes. The eyes reminded me of my father's in the year or two before his death, at eighty-two—the brightness gone from them, a certain fixed focus, as if on the far distance, or eternity. They were my eyes, all right, but they weren't looking at anything I wanted to see.

My urine bag now seemed as much a part of me as a hermit crab's shell. When I sat down, it was on the floor; when I moved from room to room, I carried it; when I lowered myself onto the bathtub seat, it was by the tub, the tube from the catheter looped over the side. I was surrounded by objects—the hand shower, the bathtub safety handles, the no-slip floor mats—that might have come straight from a catalog of old-age products, and probably had.

To a degree that I could hardly have imagined before the surgery, my body was absorbing my entire attention. To avoid the danger of embolism, I had to be careful to keep my feet propped up at all times. Anywhere I was likely to sit was covered with a rubber mat, in case of leaks, which I gradually got used to. I had supposed that once I was home I would plunge in to read through the piles of new books I had ordered, or that friends had sent me, perhaps even start doing some work—Richard, as I said, had installed extensions next to any place where I might sit, so I could connect my laptop—and reconnect myself with the office, and the world at large—but I had no desire to try it. Even *The New York Times* didn't interest me: world events, politics, reviews, I couldn't have cared less, although, to Margaret's annoyance, I *did* read the obituaries every day, to see who had died of prostate cancer (an average of about five a week in the *Times*) and to gloat over people who had died at a younger age than mine. It would be difficult to imagine an activity more suited to old age than that, as Margaret pointed out, and I could not disagree.

Every morning Margaret woke me with a cup of herbal tea—the first of the seemingly endless cups of hot and cold beverages I would drink during the day to keep my liquid intake high—then I struggled through my small routine, counting it a triumph if I could get myself shaved and brush my teeth so that I was ready for Emory and Laura, who usually arrived, separately, before eight. Once my vital signs had been taken, the nurse left and Emory helped me take my morning shower bath. Then, with Margaret and Emory's help, I got dressed. Once I was bundled up against the cold, we went for our walk. Afterward, I emptied my catheter bag again, cleaned myself up, and rested until lunchtime—my appetite had not returned, and it was all I could do to drink a cup of soup. Emory left after lunch, and I usually took an afternoon nap on the sofa in my office, then tea with Margaret, then a light supper, a little television, and it was time to clean myself up again and prepare for bed. A rich, full day. I didn't actually add up the number of hours I slept, but it was considerable—at least eight or nine hours at night, plus three or four during the day. My body seemed to know how much sleep it needed, and when it was tired it was as if a switch were simply turned off—my eyes closed and I was out like a light.

—⁂—

I HAD SET myself the task of thanking everybody who had called, written a note, or sent flowers, not just out of gratitude and good manners, but also because it seemed like something I could probably do in short spurts. I lay on my office couch, wrote cards, and made the occasional telephone call. Margaret was concerned that I not overdo it, but there was no danger of that. When I got tired, I simply stopped, sometimes in midsentence. There was no way I could have overdone anything, even if I'd wanted to.

What interested me more was a number of people who *hadn't* called or written, not, as I was to discover, because they didn't care about me, but because they simply couldn't bring themselves to face the subject of cancer. If there is any proof needed of just how much this disease is feared, it is here, among well-educated, intelligent men and women who can't even bring themselves to *say* the "c-word." One old friend sent me a paperback of inspirational poems with a note to say that he was sorry he hadn't called—that he himself was so terrified of prostate cancer he had been absolutely unable to deal with my having it. A couple we had known well for years, neighbors, went unheard from, to my surprise, until finally Margaret confronted them and asked what the matter was. They too, it turned out, couldn't deal with cancer. It was partly the fact that *I* had it—I seemed to have a certain reputation for invulnerability, or at least good luck, among my friends, thus my having cancer sent out, to some, the unhappy thought that if I of all people could get cancer, anybody could. But much more of their fear seemed to be of the disease itself, as if you could protect yourself from it by never mentioning its name.

The more people were obsessed with their own health and spiritual well-being, I discovered, the more likely they were to be unable to deal with the subject of cancer. It was as if they wanted to believe that if you did the right things and really *believed* in them, it couldn't happen to you. Since I had always kept my weight down, didn't smoke or drink to excess, ate healthily, took vitamins, and exercised regularly, I provided a frightening suggestion that none of this might matter, that what was at issue here was merely bad luck, a rogue gene rampaging around the DNA pool—plain, ordinary, dumb rotten luck.

Those who really believed in all the New Age variations of "mind over matter" didn't even want to *think* about cancer, in fact. If you believed that negative thoughts made you ill, then thoughts about cancer were like a breach in the mind's defenses. After all, cancer was about the most potent negative thought you could have. Better to pretend that it didn't exist, that it couldn't happen, to *Om* it away.

But cancer can't be *Om*'ed away, and in a great many cases it can't be rationally explained away, either. It strikes good people and bad people, vegetarians and red-meat eaters, the health-conscious and couch potatoes alike. Of course, it's always better to be fit, to eat right, to reduce stress, but with cancer there are no guarantees, and that alone is enough to scare people, even if the disease itself weren't so awful. I understood this, and therefore understood why certain people couldn't face it, and didn't hold it against them. Everybody has his or her own way of dealing with the big fears of life, and who am I, after all, to criticize those who stick their heads in the sand like the proverbial ostrich? The only thing is, I don't think it works. Ignoring cancer won't make it go away. I said as much to those friends who hadn't reached out to me because of their own fears. Margaret said a good deal more.

—⁓—

IN THE WEEKS before Christmas, I began to have visitors, for the first time since the Offits and Rod Barker had come to visit me at Johns Hopkins. I received visitors like a Turkish pasha, reclining on my office sofa in a dressing gown, with my urine bag discreetly hidden by a towel. I found that I enjoyed company, though there was no question that I tired easily. I was also, as Margaret pointed out, quick to dominate the conversation with the prostate-cancer equivalent of war stories, as if it were the only possible subject of conversation. I had to admit that this was true, but it seemed beyond me to correct it. My cancer and my surgery loomed so large in my mind that it was hard for me to think (or talk) about anything else. I would be well into the process of recovery before I could stop myself from telling people all about my health—and, not infrequently, telling them more about incontinence and impotence than they wanted to know.

The problem was that cancer, like war, is such a big event in anybody's life that it tends to blot out everything else for a long time. When visitors talked about work, movies, whatever was going on in the world, I listened with puzzlement, as if none of it made sense. It was a relief to talk to a fellow cancer patient instead, like our friend Dot Burnett, whose gentle patience I am deeply grateful for—especially since she had troubles of her own. Not even Christmas really made any sense to me, except for the fact that right after the Christmas holidays I was scheduled to have my Foley catheter removed.

That was the thing that interested me the most, the first big step on the way back to normal life. Although I was desperately afraid of what it would be like—reports were mixed from those who had experienced it, ranging from "It's a snap" to "It was the worst moment of my life"—it couldn't come a day too soon for me, and if Dr. Leslie Josephy, the Poughkeepsie urologist who had agreed to take charge of my case, and who would remove the catheter, had told me that he was going to come down the chimney Christmas Eve to remove it, it would have been the best Christmas present I had ever had.

20

As IT TURNED OUT, DR. JOSEPHY MIGHT WELL HAVE BEEN CAST IN that role. He was stout, with a grizzled silver beard and pink cheeks; he would have looked fine in a Santa Claus suit, except for his eyes, which, behind small, old-fashioned wire-rimmed glasses, were sharp and exacting—the eyes of a surgeon, in fact. He typically dressed in faded blue jeans, work boots, and a tattered work shirt, and bore some resemblance to the kind of guys you used to see around working as electricians at Grateful Dead concerts, always handy with a roll of duct tape and quick to offer you a joint. And despite his reputation as a fine surgeon, he had a workman's hands, big, with strong, blunt fingers. Dr. Josephy was, in fact, the polar opposite of Dr. Walsh: rumpled, slightly profane, and informal. He was joviality itself, as cheerful as any Santa Claus.

Although his bookshelves, I couldn't help noticing, contained two editions of Dr. Walsh's multivolume textbook on urology, Dr. Josephy turned out to be something less than an uncritical admirer of his colleague.

He studied my file briefly, reviewing the material Dr. Walsh had sent from Johns Hopkins. His expression was skeptical, even slightly derisive, as I filled him in on my experiences so far. "Nerve-sparing," he said impatiently, "what's so great about that? We all do the same operation. When I can save the nerve bundles, I do. We all do. There's no magic to it."

He looked at Dr. Walsh's notes again. "Anyway, I don't see that he's such a hotshot. He didn't save both your nerve bundles, did he? I see here he could only save one of them."

"He *didn't*?"

I was startled. This was the first news I'd had that Dr. Walsh hadn't succeeded in saving both nerve bundles! I recalled reading that when *both* nerve bundles are spared, 20 percent of men in their fifties will be impotent after surgery; when only *one* nerve bundle is spared, that figure rises to 40 percent, or a little less than half—not such hot odds, when you think about it, which I suddenly found myself doing.*

Was he *sure*? I asked Dr. Josephy, hoping he'd made a mistake.

He was sure. There it was in black and white in Dr. Walsh's notes:

> Initially the right neurovascular bundle was beautifully preserved. On the left side the bundle was also preserved, but when I took out the specimen I wanted to see a little bit more tissue back at the base, so I excised the portion of bundle adjacent to it, although residual bundle was left on the left side as well.

"I'd have probably have done the same thing," Dr. Josephy said. "The idea is to get rid of the cancer, after all. That's number one. I realize Walsh makes a big deal about sparing the nerve bundles, and that's why so many guys go to him, but that's all PR. When it comes right down to it, cancer is his number one concern, too, not saving the nerves."

I knew that, but I was still thunderstruck that nobody had ever mentioned that I had lost one nerve bundle, or most of it. "He never told me," I said.

"You probably never asked him."

That was true. I felt like an idiot for not having asked, but I still thought Dr. Walsh ought to have volunteered this information, and said so.

* These figures are from *The Prostate,* by Patrick C. Walsh, M.D., and Janet Farrar Worthington, Johns Hopkins University Press.

Josephy sighed. "Who knows? Maybe I wouldn't have told you, either. If you start getting erections again, you're a happy man, right? You didn't need to know whether you have one nerve bundle or two, did you? Anyway, that's the story. Don't let it worry you. Most men do fine, one bundle or two, and if you don't, there are plenty of things we can do to help."

I could guess what they were—the illustrations in Dr. Rous's book remained vivid in my memory, though when I had first seen them they were of merely academic interest. Dr. Josephy's enthusiasm was obvious: implants were state-of-the-art urology. Still, when people complain about Western medicine, this is exactly the kind of thing they have in mind, even if they don't know it. First you remove the patient's prostate, a brutally invasive piece of surgery; when that renders him impotent, you solve the problem by surgically implanting two inflatable paired cylinders in the shaft of his penis, linked by several feet of plastic tubing to a balloon near his bladder and a squeeze pump in his scrotum, by means of which he can transfer fluid from the balloon reservoir to the cylinders, thus producing an erection. A bypass in the scrotum allows him to deflate the whole contraption after sex, unlike the less sophisticated (and cheaper) semirigid one, which you can bend up and down like a child's toy, but which never detumesces totally, so that wearing tight jeans or a bathing suit is an embarrassment. . . .

Nothing, I thought, could persuade me to have a semirigid penile prosthesis installed, let alone the even more invasive and ambitious inflatable one. On the other hand, how would I feel a year from now, or two? It didn't look to me as if Margaret was in any mood just at the moment to hear about the wonders that Dr. Josephy could perform with surgical implants, so I headed him off at the pass.

I was still turning all this over, rather unhappily, in my mind, as Dr. Josephy summoned me into an examination room, filled a syringe to deflate the balloon in my bladder that had given me so much trouble, and said "Hold your breath." I held it, felt a slight but by no means disagreeable tug, and asked if he was about to pull the catheter out. "It's out," he said, and held it up for me to see. I expected to faint at the sight of it, but it was nothing, just a long plastic tube with what looked like a small valve at one end.

The news that I had only one nerve bundle—and the fact that I hadn't been told—upset me so much that I hadn't even noticed the removal of the catheter. I stood there, trying to get used to the absence of the catheter and its heavy urine bag.

"You're leaking on the floor," Dr. Josephy said. He didn't seem to mind. In urology, urine on the floor was normal.

I looked down. He was right. I was standing in a small pool of urine.

"Did you bring a diaper with you?"

I remembered that Emory, with his usual foresight, had put one in his pocket. With his help I struggled into my first pair of Depends Adult Incontinence Pants. They were an unfetching pale pastel green, and somewhat bulkier than I had hoped, with three sticky tabs of tape on either side to hold them in place. Emory adjusted them to his satisfaction, and I pulled my trousers over them.

"That's it," Dr. Josephy said briskly. "Keep in touch."

On the way back to the house, I could feel that my Depends were wet. I told Emory. He thought about this for a moment, obviously calculating how long the one package I had laid in before going down to Baltimore was going to last. "Better pull in here," he said, as we approached John's Apothecary.

We went home with the trunk of the car full of Depends.

I didn't know it at the time—I was still traumatized by the news about my missing nerve bundle, not to speak of my first view in so long of the world through the windshield of a car—but it was a portent of things to come.

—⁂—

SAYING GOOD-BYE TO the Foley catheter changed a lot of things, most of them for the better, but also made it clear, if I had ever had any doubts, that I was in that unhappy minority of men who experience "severe to total incontinence" after a radical prostatectomy (2 to 5 percent, according to Dr. Rous—good enough odds, if you're a betting man).

I had stubbornly assumed that I wouldn't end up with that problem, despite the leaking catheter. Emory, on the other hand, didn't seem surprised. He had looked after plenty of men in my condition. Most of them had problems with incontinence, he said, whatever the surgeons might say, and in his opinion (which he had tactfully concealed from me), men who experienced a lot of leakage around the catheter were invariably incontinent at first. I guessed Emory probably knew what he was talking about. After all, none of the urologists went home with the patient, or stuck around after the catheter was removed—besides, why give the patient bad news about what might happen when he already had plenty of other problems to handle?

Within the first twenty-four hours of the removal of the catheter, I went through a dozen Depends. John's Apothecary had only small and large in stock, but we had taken them anyway rather than run out—wisely, as it turned out, for everybody in the county seemed to be either larger or smaller than me; there were no mediums anywhere. I ordered six packages, and in the meantime made do with what I had, either squeezing myself into the small size or taping the large ones as tightly as I could so they didn't fall off. At night, I got up to change at least three times, sometimes four, and when I did, the Depends were sopping wet. I had to admit that they *worked*—they certainly soaked up the urine and prevented embarrassing accidents—but I wasn't a happy camper.

From time to time I actually found myself *missing* the catheter. The more I moved about, or got up and down, the quicker my bladder emptied. When I went for a walk, for example, the Depends soon got wet—so wet that they became heavy, uncomfortable, and even more bulky. Sometimes I could stay dry—or dryish—for an hour or more if I was sitting down with my legs up, or lying down, but the moment I was up on my feet, I was wet. Dr. Walsh, in his valedictory note, had given a hint of this in predicting that continence would return in three stages. The bladder, Emory and the nurse explained patiently (they had obviously done it before), was like a bowl. When I was seated or lying down, it was turned on its side, so the urine tended to stay in it, but when I stood up the open end was inverted, as if the bowl were turned upside down, and the urine simply ran out. Ordinarily, the urethral sphincter would hold the urine back, of course, but since the sphincter was still in shock, there was simply nothing to impede the urine from flowing out when I stood up or walked around, nor would there be until the sphincter resumed its function.

The Kegel exercises, designed to strengthen the muscles that controlled the sphincter, suddenly loomed as the most important concern of my day. Unfortunately, when it came to Kegel exercises, "you pays your money and you takes your choice," as the saying goes. The pamphlet I had received from the nurse recommended doing them twenty times, three times a day, but was vague on the subject of how to do them. Dr. Rous, in his book, described exactly how to do them, but recommended doing them only six times altogether a day, with rests in between each contraction. Professor Martin seemed to feel the more, the better, and claimed to be able to do them while driving his car. A New York specialist in incontinence dismissed all this as foolish. The exercises required intense concentration, if they were being done properly, and less than sixty at a time were useless—his patients worked their way up to hundreds—and I should keep in mind that learning to *relax* the muscles was as important as tightening them—the sequence must be exact, ten seconds for each. Dr. Walsh, as I mentioned, believed that what really mattered was a strong, unimpeded flow of urine, indicating that there was no blockage of the urethra by scar tissue, and that the patient should learn to hold back the flow while standing up, and absolutely not at any other time. As for Dr. Josephy, he did not seem to feel that it mattered one way or the other—continence would return in its own sweet time, or not, as the case might be.

I opted for the program in the pamphlet, perhaps because doing twenty contractions three times a day at least seemed like a feasible goal. The trick, I soon discovered, was learning to find the muscles to begin with. Dr. Rous's advice was helpful, but it is still no easy trick to flex a muscle you can't see and over which you have no conscious control.

Dr. Rous wrote:

> There are actually two groups of muscles that are used, the first of which is around the rectum and the second around the base of the penis. The first is the muscle you tighten when you want to suddenly stop the flow of urine while you are voiding. The second of these muscle groups is the one you would use when you think you are through voiding and want to expel the last few drops or the last "squirt" of urine. These two groups of muscles should be contracted sequentially, starting with the one you would use to stop the flow of urine while voiding and then, while keeping that muscle contracted, additionally contracting the muscle you would use to get out the last "squirt" of urine at the end of voiding. You should contract and hold in a contracted state—as tightly as you can—both these sets of muscles for ten seconds. . . .

Like a great many things that involve the involuntary muscles, this advice, detailed and specific as it may be, is far easier to read than to follow. Among the benefits of having the catheter removed was that I could now take a bath—actually lie in the water, for the first time in four weeks, instead of perching on a plastic tub chair—and I took my morning bath as an opportunity to do the day's first set of Kegel exercises. I would lie in the tub in the morning, eyes tightly closed, trying to isolate the two sets of muscles, and keeping in mind the advice from the pamphlet that if at any time you felt yourself tightening your stomach muscles you had it wrong. I had it wrong a lot of the time. It wasn't just that I wasn't doing the exercises right—I wasn't sure that I was doing them at all.

Even Emory wasn't any help. He couldn't see the two muscle groups any more than I could, after all. I flexed and released fiercely, hoping I was doing some good, but no matter how many Kegel exercises I performed, I still had no substantial control over urination. Maybe the only good thing about it was that lying in a tub full of hot water was about the most comfortable thing I could do. It wasn't just that a bath is soothing—I felt a strong need to bathe inspired by a fear that I smelled of urine, even though this wasn't actually true. Besides, cradled softly in the water, I felt restored to humanity again. If I voided urine, it went unseen and unnoticed. From time to time, I made myself look at the incision, a thick red line now, with the punctures from the staples and the drains fading away. My pubic hair was beginning to grow back, but my genitals were still shrunken. I had been assured that this was par for the course, but it still wasn't a sight that gave me any pleasure.

Even had I wanted to follow Dr. Walsh's advice about holding back the flow of urine, there was no way I could get to a bathroom in time to follow it. When the urge to urinate came on, it was usually impossible to resist, a problem made more acute by the fact that most of my time downstairs was spent in my study, a long way from the nearest toilet, which was up a steep flight of narrow, uneven, eighteenth-century stairs. There was simply no way I could swing my legs off the sofa—I was still obliged to keep them up as much as possible—get to my feet, and creep up the stairs while trying to keep my sphincter clenched. Mostly, I failed.

At the nurse's suggestion, I evolved a different method. She sent Emory off to buy a few male urinals, the plastic receptacles with handles, wide necks, and covers, with which anybody who has ever been in a hospital will be familiar. We placed one in the small alcove off my study. We placed another next to my side of the bed. Now, all I had to do was to make it a few feet to the alcove, if I was downstairs, or simply stand up, if I was in bed, then pee into the urinal, trying to interrupt the flow as often as possible, just as Dr. Walsh suggested.

It worked. At first I was unable to hold the flow back at all; soon I could hold it back for a few seconds at a time at will, even when my bladder was full. I saw, for the first time, a ray of hope. Perhaps even more important, from the psychological point of view at least, I was no longer peeing in my pants. It wasn't much fun making a rush for the urinal and trying to hold back the urine until I could get to it (let alone getting my trousers unzipped, my Depends unstuck—the six sticky adhesive closing tapes were not ideally suited for speedy disrobing—and pulled down, which didn't always work out in time, alas), but as the flow started I felt a glow of satisfaction, for I was in control again, however tentative and precarious, of my own urinary system.

The downside was that my bladder, recovering from surgery, had altogether its own sense of timing and measurement. I had to get up and use the urinal constantly, sometimes as often as every fifteen minutes, for the bladder signaled, with treacherous urgency, that it was full when, in fact, it contained only a few ounces of urine. I could not resist its urgent signal to void even when I knew, intellectually, that it was a false alarm. Even so, I had made a step forward, a bigger one than I knew, for the sensations I was feeling, however trying, were a sign that nerves and tissue had survived the assault, were gradually reawakening. They might be producing mixed signals, and there was no guarantee that they would ever return to what they had been before surgery, but at least they were not dead. Healing was a possibility.

—⁓—

THERE WERE OTHER signs of healing. Though I had been showered with gifts of food and delicacies, and the Bacons had stocked every cupboard in the house with things to eat, I had not really felt any hunger at all since the operation. Then, one afternoon, while I was sitting in the kitchen with Richard Bacon and Emory, Richard happened to mention that he was going to Sunny's, our local sandwich shop–deli, to get something for lunch. Would I like anything? he asked. I thought about it. Yes, I said, I would like a BLT on rye toast, with ketchup, no mayo. Richard gave a grin, and returned soon with not one, but *two,* BLTs, and I ate them both as if I were starving. They tasted better than anything I had ever eaten in the best restaurants of Paris.

A few days later, Margaret said to me, "Let's go out to dinner." I was startled—scared by the suggestion, frankly. Except for my daily walk and the visit to Dr. Josephy, I had not been out of the house since my return from Johns Hopkins. The very idea of sitting in a car still made me nervous—somehow all my thoughts focused on the tenderness and fragility of my incision and the many cuts and stitches deep under it. What if the car skidded? What if someone else skidded and hit us? Besides, how would my bladder react to being out of the house? But Margaret clearly meant business, so I pushed my fears aside and let myself be bundled into the car and driven a mile or two to the Village Restaurant, a nearby diner, where I sat cautiously in a booth, on the foam pillow that was my constant companion now, and ate scrambled eggs and bacon with toast. Margaret had wisely picked the local diner because we could always just get up and go if I became uncomfortable, and because it was only a few minutes from home, but in the event, there were no problems. My Depends were wet when I got home, but I felt as jubilant as a prisoner released from jail.

"There's a lesson," Margaret said as we were driving back to the house, as I clutched a pillow to my incision, just in case. "Do something new every day, however small it is."

I thought about this. "No big leaps, you mean? Just a steady upward progress. Small victories?"

"I'd call tonight a big leap," Margaret said. "You got in the car and went out to dinner. But, yes, small victories is just what I mean." She turned into our driveway. "It's time we went out to the movies, is what I think."

Movies, I should explain, play a major role in our life. Margaret and I are inveterate moviegoers for whom videocassettes remain a poor second. By now, after several weeks of what was doubtless beginning to seem to Margaret like house arrest, we had had our fill of videos. There were plenty of new movies Margaret wanted to see, and she was determined to see them—with me.

That seemed like a big step to me. I could hardly take my urinal with me, and I didn't relish the thought of having to get up and go to the bathroom constantly, carrying a supply of Depends to change into with me. It was Emory who came up with the suggestion of using a "condom catheter," which I approached cautiously, given Dr. Walsh's warnings against them. Still, Dr. Walsh wasn't the one who was faced with the challenge of going out to the movies, so Emory and I went to John's Apothecary and returned with the various bits and pieces of the device, a small, transparent bag that fit to the ankle with Velcro straps, rather like a detective's ankle holster, a length of flexible tubing, and what looked exactly like a rolled condom except that it had a short tube at the end of it that mated with the end of the flexible tubing. It was a straightforward device, the modern, plastic version of what used to be called "the Brakeman's Friend," a piece of equipment used by railwaymen who couldn't leave their controls to urinate. The only major difference was that the condom part of this new contraption was a one-time-only item—once it had been unrolled onto the penis, that was it, you threw it away when you finally removed it. The rest of it could be washed in antiseptic soap and cleaned off with an alcohol pad.

I could see one problem right away. Getting the condom unrolled and secured over a flaccid penis was a challenge. The manufacturer had attempted to reduce this problem by placing a strip of adhesive on the inside of the condom, to make sure it stayed on and to produce a watertight seal between the plastic and the skin, but one's pubic hairs had a tendency to get stuck, so that taking off the condom became an exercise in self-inflicted pain. Still, I was determined to go to the movies, so I persevered.

The first time I went out with the condom catheter on I walked as if I were on eggshells, but I soon discovered that it worked reliably enough. As with the Foley catheter, you had to be careful to empty the bag before it filled—there was a handy little tap at the bottom of it for that—and there was an irresistible tendency to reach into one's trousers and make sure the condom was still on, but, of course, it always was—the trick was taking it *off*, not keeping it *on*. When sitting down, you had to make sure that the flexible tube didn't get kinked, blocking the flow.

When the great evening dawned I made my way proudly to the car, and held myself protectively as Margaret drove us to the movie theater—the longest drive I had experienced so far. I took an aisle seat, just in case (I had also stuffed a Depends in each pocket of my parka, to use if the condom catheter turned out to be a disaster), but despite a lot of nervousness on my part, there were no problems, except that I had to get up from time to time to let gravity drain the urine into the bag, and go to the bathroom twice to empty the bag, which was designed more for discretion than for quantity.

—⁂—

"ANOTHER VICTORY," MARGARET said as I got back into the car. I was exhausted, not only by emotion but also because it was the first time I had been in a crowd of people since before the surgery. I had been desperately afraid that somebody would bump into me—in fact, I carried a cane, not because I really needed one, but in order to fend people off, since it is a universally recognized and respected symbol of invalidism.

Margaret was right. It was a victory—a significant one. Soon, I was not only going to the movies, but even going out to restaurants for dinner—*real* restaurants, not diners. I could not, of course, do both in one evening as yet, but I sensed that that, too, would eventually come—dinner and a movie!

I felt a certain guilt at having breached one of Dr. Walsh's rules, but Dr. Josephy, after all, had been a fervent advocate of the condom catheter—of anything, in fact, that made incontinence more bearable. When I complained of bladder pains, he put me on Ditropan (with Dr. Walsh's approval), which stopped them at once, though it numbered among its side effects a tormenting thirst and a dry throat that made my voice even more breathless and gravelly than before. Still, it worked.

Even though the condom catheter freed me up to go out for the evening, it was not without its problems, as I soon discovered. It *was* possible for the condom to become detached, with embarrassing results, and there was no way I could wear it for more than a couple of hours at a time, for by that time the skin of the penis was raw and painful, so much so that I tried not to use the device more than once every few days, for "special" occasions like a movie or dinner with friends. At times, it backed up uncomfortably, if I was sitting down, and it was often necessary to stand up, sometimes for most of a movie.

On one occasion, the condom was the proximate cause of a terrible outburst of rage on my part. We were hurrying to get to the movies on time and I inadvertently neglected to close the small tap at the bottom of the bag. By the time I got downstairs, I realized that my slippers were wet, as well as my socks; then, to my puzzlement, I noticed that I was standing in a pool of water, that there were, in fact, drops of water all over the carpeted stairs. . . . For a moment, I couldn't make out what had happened, then I let out a howl of frustrated anger and rage. My anger was uncontrollable, a kind of pointless, self-directed rage, rage at my helplessness, rage at my humiliation (in my own eyes, for Margaret, to her credit, remained calm), rage at what had become of me. We cleaned up the floor, I changed my socks and threw away my slippers, and we went to the movies, but the accident had taught me just how fragile my self-control was.

Small things—the repeated failure of our oil company to fix the hot-water heater and the furnace, for example—sent me into soaring rages that left me shaking and in tears. What effect they had on, say, the furnace repairman I couldn't tell, but they were profoundly out of character for me. Anger, in my case, normally produces sarcasm and coldness; now it was producing truly operatic displays of temperament, in which I howled at my targets, often total strangers, "I am a cancer patient," over and over again, just to make them feel worse.

At that point I decided that the only sensible thing was to get back to work as soon as possible—I needed to reestablish control over *something*. I also started to explore the various treatments for incontinence—for I recognized that Dr. Walsh was right, as usual. The condom catheter was a pretty good way of getting out to see a movie, but it wasn't foolproof, and when it went wrong it plunged me into rage or depression—besides which, it wasn't moving me forward at all. The more you wore it, the more you needed it: it was a crutch.

There were other forms of catheter, of course. A catalog for the aging produced one which didn't use a condom; instead, it had a sort of funnel, held in place by a leather strap around the waist, into which you placed the penis. It didn't work, however, so I junked it, along with a spring-loaded device that you were supposed to place between your buttocks and squeeze, to improve the Kegel exercises, and which I couldn't even compress. I developed pains in the area of the sphincter, almost certainly from having strained the muscles, just as Dr. Walsh had warned.

There was no rushing the healing process, I decided. I went back to doing what he had suggested in the first place—stopping the flow while standing up, and nothing else. For going to dinner or the movies, I took a lot of Depends with me, and changed them whenever I needed to.

Continence would take time, I belatedly came to accept, and that was that.

21

I HAD BEEN SAILING ALONG, PRETTY MUCH IGNORING THE *REST* OF MY body, when out of the blue one day, while Margaret was shopping, I was seized with the violent stomach cramps of extreme constipation. I could neither rise, nor walk, nor pass the obstruction in my bowels.

Dr. Walsh had warned of the danger of straining the muscles while passing a stool—it was the thing that any patient recovering from a radical prostatectomy had to be most careful about.

I had been careful—or thought I had—but here I was, straining hopelessly on the toilet, in agony. Luckily, Emory was there. When he realized that I could not straighten up at all, he called an ambulance. I insisted that we had to wait for Margaret's return, since I hadn't wanted her to be alarmed by coming home and finding me gone, and she arrived with her shopping bags just as I was being loaded into the ambulance. We set off for the hospital in a convoy, me in the ambulance with Emory, and Margaret in our car with Richard Bacon.

The rest of that day was a nightmare. For hours I lay on a gurney in the emergency room while the beleaguered emergency-room staff tried everything they could to remove the blockage, including Ducolax suppositories and repeated enemas with cold water. Nothing worked until one of the doctors, either out of pity or more likely simply to shut me up, gave me an injection of Toradol, a painkiller, then dug out the impaction bit by bit. No doctor could have been kinder and more efficient than young Dr. Zale; no patient could possibly have made more of a fuss. Whatever reserves of courage or optimism I had stored up were gone. At the end of the day, I emerged from the hospital more or less on my own steam, and went home.

I had learned a valuable lesson. Without giving it much thought, I had been committing the cardinal sin of trying to control the frequency of urination by drinking less. Some urologists may suggest cutting back on the liquid intake when the patient suffers from incontinence, simply because it makes life slightly more bearable for the patient, but there is a price to pay, as usual. At the same time, they urge the patient to keep taking milk of magnesia and mineral oil, which I had gradually given up doing, since there seemed to be no need for them.

The moment my nurse heard that I was in the emergency room, she knew what had happened, and by the next morning I was on *her* regime: huge quantities of liquid, particularly herbal tea and orange juice (the kind that has bits of orange floating around it); Metamucil, a stool softener, in my juice; and a fiber intake so high that I seemed to be eating mounds of broccoli at every meal. I felt like one of those elderly retirees in certain parts of Florida who sit around the shuffleboard court in the mornings talking about laxatives, a character straight out of a Philip Roth novel.

Still, anything, even Metamucil, was better than an impaction. It was not an experience I wanted to have a second time, and so long as I kept to my high-fiber/high-liquid regime, I never had a problem again.

—m—

I THOUGHT FOR a long time about what had happened in the emergency room. I, who am usually very controlled, had what amounted to a public screaming fit during the hours I was in the emergency room. I was in pain, yes, but instead of holding the pain back, I had let it go—let it go in a long, loud, uncontrollable burst, along with a huge accumulation of frustration and fear.

It was out of character, but there had been nothing I could do to stop myself. I howled, sobbed, cried, shouted at the nurses, demanded to see the doctor, moaned, and whimpered, until finally I was given a painkiller. It was as if something had snapped in me— here I was, back in the hospital again, in the most painful and humiliating of circumstances, with no control over *anything*, unable to shit, unable to stop pissing, tangled up in a sweaty hospital gown soaked in my own urine, dragged at intervals into a cold, tiled bathroom where two nurses (plus Emory, who had cast himself as my protector) attempted to give me an ice-cold enema and failed, knowing all the time that if this *didn't* get resolved I was going to end up with a temporary colostomy bag, if not worse. Surely, I thought, I had enough problems to deal with without *this*. Surely this just wasn't *fair*.

Of course, life is *not* fair, and I knew it, just as I knew that there were plenty of people with problems far worse than my own—

however much pain I was in—some of them no doubt in the same emergency room as I, listening to my shrieks and moans. All this I knew, but for a few hours I was without shame.

That night, as I lay in bed, the pain already a fast-dimming memory, Margaret said that she had never seen me so angry.

I denied it. I wasn't angry, I told her. Frightened and in pain, yes, but surely *not* angry. After all, I had nobody to be angry *at*—my impaction wasn't anybody's fault, any more than my cancer had been anybody's fault. These things happened, that was all.

"No," Margaret said firmly. "You were angry."

She took my hand. "You have a right to be angry," she said. "I'd be angry if something like this had happened to me. So don't kid yourself. I know anger when I see it."

I had to admit that she was right. I *was* kidding myself. Anger had been boiling up in me for a long time—not just anger, but *rage*, all the harder to deal with since it wasn't directed at anybody in particular. It was rage at what had become of me, rage at the slowness of my recuperation, rage at my own helplessness. I was not angry at doctors or hospitals—I had nothing to blame them for—but I raged that the control of my life had passed, so swiftly, from my hands to theirs. It was anger fueled by the unanswerable question *"Why me?"*

I had held myself in check for nearly three months now, but Margaret was right: the anger had been there all the time, building, growing, occasionally erupting in fitful bursts of self-pity when something went wrong, and finally erupting in the emergency room like a volcano. I felt at once ashamed, relieved, and exhausted.

I was shortly to discover that I wasn't alone when it came to anger. It exists in every prostate-cancer patient, to a greater or lesser degree—even those who have been "cured."

—⁊⁊⁊—

I CAN'T SPEAK for other kinds of cancer, but prostate-cancer patients are a clubby lot, eager to share their experiences. No less than two of my neighbors turned out to be recuperating from radical prostatectomies; by coincidence both of them jogged up and down the road in front of our house every morning—I had seen them a thousand times before, when I took my morning run, and nodded or said hello without knowing their names. The sight of me staggering up the road on Emory's arm, carrying my urine bag, had prompted them to ask what had happened.

One of them, Bill, a local educator, dropped in to see me and fill me in on *his* experience with prostate cancer. *He* had been operated on locally about a year before, and seemed pleased by the result. He had had "some" incontinence, but it passed quickly, and he was now "dry," except when he laughed, or coughed, or bent down to pick up something heavy. His PSA was below 0.5—about as low as you can get—and he was back to normal when it came to work and exercise. I filled him in on my situation. Yes, he said, he had gone through some rough moments, but you turned a corner, and after that it was fine—I would find that out for myself.

I sensed there was more to it than that. Bill sat rigidly, not at all the picture of a man for whom life was back to normal again. I did not, in fact, have the impression that he had come to comfort me so much as to talk about himself. Had he recovered potency? I asked. A flash of anger crossed his face—not at me, I could tell that, but at life. Clearly, I was not the only person to ask, uselessly, *"Why me?"*

Sex was a problem—no, *the* problem. Bill had waited in vain for erections to return. Both nerve bundles had been spared, he felt like a million dollars, his wife was eager to resume sex, *but nothing happened.* His expression was grim, lips firmly compressed in anger. He clutched the teacup so hard that I was afraid he would break off the handle. His wife had tried everything, he said, but *nada*—zip. It was all very painful for both of them—worse, really, for her, he thought, because whereas he was in his early fifties, his wife was in her thirties. Luckily they had children, still . . . She had certain expectations, of course, natural in a woman her age, which weren't being met. . . .

Did she complain about that? I asked.

Bill gave me a dark, moody glare. No, he said defensively, she wasn't the type who complained. She had never raised the subject, in fact. . . . But he could *tell* . . . He had made up his mind what to do, however. He was going to have the implant. He had discussed it with his urologist, and was determined to go ahead as soon as possible.

"What does your wife think about that?" I asked.

"She'll be delighted. Why wouldn't she be?"

"Whoa!" I said. "You mean you haven't *talked* to her about it?"

Bill saw no reason to talk to her about it. It was his problem, not hers, and it was up to him to get it solved, he said stubbornly—*angrily*, in fact.

I did not want to give offense—and it was surely none of my business—but I knew he was wrong. How could he *possibly* know what his wife wanted? I asked him. Maybe she was content with things the way they were. Some women might even be glad, or relieved. There were other options, anyway, even if she was unhappy, without going blindly into an invasive piece of surgery that involved inevitable complications, who knew what side effects and how much pain, and which was irreversible—for once the implant was in, you were stuck with it. Why not take it by stages, starting with the least invasive methods? He should surely at least *consider* the alternatives: injections that could stimulate an erection, a vacuum pump, all sorts of things, not to mention that there were all sorts of sexual relations you could have without an erection. . . .

I realized I was spouting a combination of wishful thinking and information picked up from reading Dr. Rous's book and articles by and about Dr. Walsh—besides which, I wasn't a sex therapist, after all—but the idea of Bill's deciding to plunge straight into a surgical implant without sitting down and discussing it with his wife struck me as loony, and I said so. It was as if the responsibility for "sex," however that was defined, was entirely his, and that everything would be "solved" once he had an erection, by however artificial (and intrusive) a means.

He went away unconvinced. Bill had come, ostensibly, to make *me* feel better, and instead I had merely made him feel worse. His anger had been palpable, like a kind of aura, though he had it firmly under control. I did not like to imagine what would happen if the implant, once he had it, didn't work as expected, or if his wife wasn't as pleased with it as he expected her to be. Would he not then blame her for failing to appreciate what he had gone through on her behalf? Giving a man an implant that would produce an erection at will for as long as he wanted after a year of impotence might cause more problems than it solved. It was, I thought, a mechanistic, plumber's answer to a question that involved so many complex needs, emotions, and habits, and that most people barely understood in the first place.

I thought about my own situation, too. What I had told Bill was what I told myself in the middle of the night. Did I really believe it? Yes, absolutely. But would I still feel the same a year after surgery, if I was still impotent (or, as Dr. Josephy preferred to put it, "suffering from erectile dysfunction")? I didn't know the answer to that, and I hoped I wouldn't have to find out.

—⁊⁊⁊—

ANOTHER NEIGHBOR, ELLIOTT, was more reticent about sex. *His* problems were of a different nature. He had undergone surgery for a radical prostatectomy about eighteen months before, and the operation had been successful—or had seemed to be, until his PSA, which had dropped to almost 0, zoomed back up to 9. Now he was trying to decide what to do. His urologist advised radiation, but he had sought a second opinion and been advised to try hormone therapy. His HMO would not cover the second opinion, however, so he was out what it had cost him as well as stuck with two different recommendations, and not at all sure which to follow. . . . Besides, he was retired; he couldn't afford to go on hormones if his insurance company wouldn't cover them. In the meantime, he said, eyes flashing with anger—though he seemed the mildest of men—he felt fine, he had recovered completely. His incontinence had been difficult, sure, but it was gone now, except during the occasional stress, lifting and carrying, and so on. He jogged two miles every day, enjoyed life, everything was back to normal, better than normal, in fact, *but he still had cancer, and nobody could offer him a good, clear explanation of what to do about it.* His was the simple anger of a man who couldn't get a straight story and who felt that he was being jerked around by the insurance establishment.

I suggested that he buy Dr. Rous's book, and perhaps *Choices: Realistic Alternatives in Cancer Therapy* as well, but beyond that I could only listen sympathetically. That, however, is what matters most, as I was beginning to learn. None of us is an oncologist, or a urologist, but they are not always good listeners—most doctors simply don't have the time. Wives, friends, siblings, parents, professional therapists, may all be good listeners, but they haven't lived through it, they simply don't *know* what it's like. . . . But those who *have* been through it *understand*—understand about impotence, incontinence, the fear of waiting to hear what the number is after a PSA test, the difficulty of getting straight answers out of doctors, and the occasional pain of getting a straighter answer than you wanted.

So I listened, just as he would listen to me the next time our paths crossed as we took our exercise. I never got to know him well, in the conventional sense of friendship, or Bill either, but I could and did tell both of them intimate things about my life that I would have found hard to share with my closest friends, and they could do the same with me. Talking to them helped me to deal with my anger. My own problems seemed to fall into perspective when I spoke to Bill and Elliott, and I learned all sorts of things from them, from practical tips for dealing with stress incontinence—carry a Maxipad in your pocket and slip it into your Jockey shorts—to the bigger issues of dealing with family, employers, and the world at large. I did not have Bill's problem, for instance—an employer who effectively wrote him off the moment Bill let it be known he had cancer—or Elliott's, which was the difficulty of getting his insurer to pay for the kind of treatment he thought he needed or the consultation he wanted, and struggling to make up the difference on a retirement budget. Cancer is never good news, but for a lot of people it is made more frightening by just such considerations: Your boss may jump to the conclusion that you're going to be out of the office a lot, and may not make it in the long run, so why not give that promotion to a younger, healthier man. Your insurance company or HMO, smelling the possibility of major claims, may prove inflexible and uncooperative about your choice of doctor or hospital. Family members may either drown you with sympathy or give you none.

The first thought of a lot of men upon being told they have prostate cancer is not "I'm going to die" but "I'm going to lose my job." The second thought, all too often, is "Will my medical insurance cover all of it?"—and, shortly after that, "Will I be able to choose the doctor I trust—and how do I know if I can trust him?"

There are no easy answers to such questions. A lot of companies pay lip service to supporting an employee through his cancer treatment until he's back to work again, but for many men cancer is the kiss of death, so far as their careers are concerned. As for medical insurance, there are horror stories galore about people who found that their coverage ran out long before their treatment did, or who couldn't get the doctor—or the second opinion, or the treatment—that they wanted unless they paid for it out of pocket, which they couldn't afford, particularly when the cancer has metastasized to the bone and you're talking about strontium 89 injections at several thousand dollars apiece. Elliott's situation, for instance, was nothing like as dire as that, but still, his insurance company wanted him to stick with his present doctor while what *he* wanted to do was to make a choice. When you think your life may be at stake—or at the very least, your capacity to enjoy what remains of it for as long as possible—that's enough to make you angry.

22

IT WAS THROUGH ELLIOTT THAT I LEARNED ABOUT THE LOCAL prostate-cancer support group that met twice a month in the American Cancer Society's building on the grounds of Vassar Brothers Hospital in Poughkeepsie. I hadn't even *heard* of it, I told him (besides which, I left unsaid, I'm not good at that kind of thing). The next day a flier was left in my mailbox. There was no doubt in my mind that I had plenty of questions about my recuperation that weren't being answered by my urologists, so despite my reservations, I decided to go to the next meeting. Dr. Josephy was skeptical. He wasn't sure it would help me—it might even depress me. A lot of grousing went on at these meetings, he said, and his expression suggested that much of it was probably directed at doctors.

Emory took me there (his presence was to give rise to the rumor that I was accompanied everywhere by a bodyguard). We had debated the matter, and decided that since the meeting ran from seven P.M. to nine, I would be more comfortable wearing my condom catheter. In one corner of a large auditorium about thirty middle-aged and older men huddled around a big table; I couldn't help wondering how many of them were similarly outfitted. My first reaction as I signed in was that most of the men looked pretty fit, despite their disease (and their age)—nobody, at any rate, was in a wheelchair or using a walker. My next reaction was that prostate cancer clearly cuts across all the socioeconomic and racial boundaries. There were several black men (blacks, as it happens, have by far the highest rate of prostate cancer in the United States—nobody knows why yet); several men in well-cut suits; quite a few blue-collar workers wearing jackets with union logos on the back or the names of the companies they worked for; a lot of men who had the casually dressed look of retirees; guys who looked like car salesmen; guys who had the unmistakable look of teachers or college professors—in short, as democratic a cross section as you could possibly ask for. Prostate cancer was clearly an equal-opportunity disease.

The atmosphere was relaxed, even clubby. Except for the absence of a bar and the uncompromising signs forbidding smoking, it might have been the meeting of a social club. As in any club, there was a distinct division between the regulars who knew each other well and had staked out seats at the table and the newcomers seated nervously behind them on metal folding chairs. The regulars all had thick briefcases or file folders on the table in front of them, stuffed with charts, letters, X rays, correspondence—their whole case histories, down to the last detail. On the blackboard somebody had written, in a clear hand, "Knowledge = Survival!"

Promptly at seven, the group's leader, a wiry, healthy-looking man in his fifties, brought the meeting to order. Dennis O'Hara had founded the group when he discovered that he couldn't get answers to his own questions after a radical prostatectomy, and that there were no support groups for men with prostate cancer.* He asked the first-timers to introduce themselves. When it was my turn, I rose. I said that I had had a radical prostatectomy performed at Johns Hopkins (several Johns Hopkins alumni nodded) by Dr. Patrick Walsh (a

---

* The first prostate-cancer group was founded by a prostate-cancer survivor named James F. Mullen in Sarasota, Florida, in 1989, after Mullen found that the only cancer support groups available were for men and women, and usually run by women. Most men, he realized, were unable to talk frankly about incontinence and impotence in front of women, or to use "locker room language" in which to describe their problems. ("I didn't want to hear about their cervix and they didn't want to hear about my prostate," as one member put it.) The idea of an all-male group "just kind of mushroomed," as Mullen says, and there are hundreds today, some of them called Man to Man, after the original one. Most groups invite wives and significant others at regular intervals, usually to hear a guest speaker, and there is now a group for them, too, called Side by Side. Meetings are invariably held under the auspices of the local American Cancer Society. The people there are always happy to provide information about the meetings, which are open to anybody who has or thinks he may have prostate cancer.

few admiring whistles—Dr. Walsh's name was one to conjure with here), who said he had removed all the cancer ("We've heard that one before," somebody whispered at the far end of the table). I was recuperating pretty well, I added, except for incontinence, which I was finding very hard to take. I had put on a condom catheter to come to this meeting, but even when it worked properly, which wasn't always the case, I didn't like or trust the device.

Dennis counted the weeks since my Foley catheter had been removed quickly on his fingers, and gave a quick laugh. "It's been three *weeks*," he said. "Start worrying in three *months*, why don't you, man?" A laugh went around the table. It was not unfriendly. On the contrary, it was warm, hearty, genial laughter—everybody there had been where I was at one time, and understood the way I felt. Welcome to the club. Perhaps because I had been frank about the subject, one of the older regulars made room for me to squeeze my chair in at the table. "You'll see, kid," he said, as if I were his grandchild, instead of sixty-one to his seventy or so, "it'll work out. Hell, if the worst that happens is you piss in your pants a little every once in a while, you're a lucky man."

This was the only place I had been where confessing to incontinence produced laughter. The thought was comforting, even consoling. We were all in this together, knights of the Maxipad and the condom catheter. Some of the older members, now that I was at the table and looking at them more closely, did not actually look so hot. The man sitting on the other side of me shook my hand with a firm grip. He was old—certainly more than seventy—bald, his face darkly tanned, lined, and seamy, like an old, worn-out piece of leather, and his teeth had the square, regular, porcelain look of dentures. "My PSA is 200," he whispered to me proudly in a gravelly baritone, "the highest in the group."

A PSA that high hardly seemed possible to me,* but he had already slipped me a Xerox copy of the lab report, on which, high-

---

* Later, I would discover that my new acquaintance was wrong about holding the record. One man in the group had a PSA of 400; another, 800!

lighted in fluorescent pink, I could read his noteworthy score. I handed it back to him with a nod of thanks. "That's ten years after a radical prostatectomy," he whispered. Then: "I'm seventy-nine, and me and the missus just came back from a world cruise, so you see?" I saw, all right. Incontinence three weeks after the removal of my Foley catheter paled into insignificance beside this man's having survived for ten years with a PSA in the *Guinness Book of Records* class.

Dennis wasn't through with me yet, however. How much did I really know about my cancer? Not much, it turned out, as the regulars chuckled at my ignorance. Did I know the dimensions of my tumor, how many grams it was, exactly where it had been sited? Did I have my pathology reports? I did not. Knowledge, Dennis said, equaled survival. I was entitled to all my records. Doctors tried to hold on to them, they behaved as if the records were *their* property, not yours, but if—God forbid—my cancer recurred, my life might depend on how much information I had about my case. My records were my lifeline, and I should never forget that. (Dennis, I noticed, had beside him on the table a giant briefcase, overflowing with his case history in neatly cross-indexed files.)

There was a lot of nodding of heads at this comment. Here, the omniscient wisdom of doctors was not, it appeared, a given. Most of these people had become self-taught experts on prostate cancer, Dennis more than any. The doctors, Dennis said, had tunnel vision. If they did radical prostatectomies, then that was what they knew about and recommended, ditto the radiologists. Besides which, they were busy men—they were not all like Pat Walsh; they didn't necessarily have the time (or the inclination) to read up on the latest medications or procedures—and they were inclined to dismiss anything new or unfamiliar as dangerous hogwash. They didn't know what was happening in Europe, they weren't following the latest studies—in short, you, the patient, had to tell *them,* the doctors, what was going on out there in the world beyond their own offices or operating rooms, and then overcome their hostility and resistance.

Leaflets were being passed around the room to newcomers. One was from the National Coalition for Cancer Survivorship (NCCS), and listed "the Cancer Survivor's Bill of Rights" (briefly summed up, this centered on "the right to assurance of lifelong medical care," "the right to the pursuit of happiness," "equal job rights," and "health insurance," all of which were put at risk when a person developed cancer). The other was from PAACT, Inc. (Patient Advocates for Advanced Cancer Treatments), an organization dedicated to making cancer patients more aware of the details of their own cases—the cover of their flier bore this advice: "You are in charge of your own destiny. Throughout your treatment, you will enlist the services of a team of physicians, but remember: it is your life that is at stake. The decisions to be made are yours!" PAACT provided a case-history form that ran to nine densely packed pages of questions, none of which, to my shame, I could answer.

"Who's in charge?" Dennis asked, pointing at me accusingly.

"I am," I said rather tentatively. There was a round of applause, rather lukewarm, so I had obviously guessed the right answer.

"And who are you?"

That one stumped me. Clearly, the answer was not "Michael Korda." I made a guess. "A cancer victim?"

There was a howl of derision and dismay from around the table, which Dennis masterfully silenced. I did not know what he actually did in private life, but he would have made a fine prosecutor in a tribunal of the French Revolution. I felt like Sidney Carton in *A Tale of Two Cities.*

"No," he said, delighted that I had provided the occasion for driving home another lesson. "Are we *victims?*" he asked.

The men around the table shook their heads and muttered "No." Dennis was clearly in charge here—probably no group like this ever succeeds unless it develops a leader who devotes his full-time attention to it—but like his members, for the most part, he had been made gentle and caring by the shared experience with cancer.

"A cancer survivor," Dennis said, facing me. "Never forget that. *You are NOT a victim!* You're a *survivor.* A victim is somebody who's helpless, who has no control over his own fate. You're not helpless. Your fate is in your hands. Got it?"

"Got it," I said.

He reached over and shook my hand—a hearty, firm handshake, conferring, as I instantly understood, full membership in the group. I had let myself be used in good spirits as an object lesson for the other newcomers. It was a rite of initiation, of sorts, and when I sat down, the two older men on either side of me patted me on the shoulder.

I looked a little more closely at the NCCS material, and understood, very quickly, why the anger around this table went beyond the subject of doctors. Cancer survivors ("a new minority of eight million Americans" that I had just joined) often became medically uninsurable if their illness went on long enough, unless they were taken on by state-mandated risk pools or open enrollment programs, both of which were threatened by reduced funding and new health-care legislation at both the federal and the state levels. Cancer survivors were often discriminated against in the workplace, stigmatized socially, and, in those cases where pain was an issue, provided with inadequate relief or made to feel guilty because they demanded medication strong enough to enable them to function.

I had not experienced any of these phenomena myself, as yet, and hoped not to, but even I could understand what the NCCS (and Dennis) were talking about. People who have had cancer *are* treated as a kind of minority group, as if the most important thing about them is their cancer, much as many people still treat African Americans, as if the only thing that matters about them (or to them) is that they are black. And I had seen myself, in the past, how quickly people wrote off a colleague or a subordinate with cancer, offering a degree of sympathy while at the same time taking it for granted that the person involved probably wasn't going to be around for very long.

("Larry would be perfect for the job." "I hear he has cancer." "He *does*? Poor guy. . . . You know, Sam would probably be pretty good for the job, too, now that I think of it.") And yet, as the NCCS pointed out, of the eight million American cancer survivors, no less than *four* million have lived productively with their diagnosis for five years or more. About half of the nation's cancer patients have been returned by modern medical advances to their normal life span (59 percent for those under fifty-five years old). That's a lot of cancer survivors out there living, or *trying* to live, normal lives.

The other newcomers were introducing themselves now. The first was a tall, muscular black man, very good-looking, in his early forties, with an engaging smile. He had been diagnosed with prostate cancer, he told us, and had carefully considered all the alternatives. He had decided against having a radical prostatectomy, and chosen cryoablation instead, which he had had a year ago, and his PSA was way down. This fascinated me. In all the books I had read, cryoablation, a new and experimental technique of freezing the prostate tissue to kill the tumors, was dismissed as unproven and dangerous, even outlandish, yet here was a healthy-looking man who had undergone the procedure with apparent success. Had he had any incontinence? I asked. He shook his head. None at all. And impotence? He laughed gently. No, he said, that was the reason he had chosen cryoablation in the first place. He had learned there was a risk of impotence from surgery, and he was just not about to take that risk. He was—he had to admit it—something of a ladies' man. There was no doubt about it, he said, he liked the ladies all right, and they liked *him,* if we got his meaning.

We got his meaning, all right. I detected a somewhat uncharitable feeling around the table, perhaps because the rest of us were being confronted with an African American man who was proudly confirming a well-known white belief about black male sexuality—or perhaps most of these men were struggling with reduced libido from hormone treatments or "erectile dysfunction" from surgery or radiation. Even if he had been white, he would not have made a lot of friends in this group by saying that he was a ladies' man.

In any event, he had been well-satisfied by the procedure, which had been quick and relatively pain-free. The probe was inserted, the cancer was frozen, and that was that. His sex life had been totally unaffected, and his PSA was down from 15 to 3. He was a happy man.

I could see Dennis struggling with his feelings. On the one hand, he did not want to throw cold water over this man's enthusiasm for cryoablation, particularly since he had had the procedure and there was no going back for him—and probably no going forward, if there was a problem, since cryoablation would very likely have ruled out future surgery. On the other hand, a PSA of 3 *after* the procedure was not necessarily good news. It could mean that there were still cancer cells present, and that the cryoablation should have been followed up with hormone therapy or radiation. After a radical prostatectomy, or successful radiation, the PSA should drop down to nearly 0, or as near as possible. My admiration for Dennis grew when he gently suggested that he wanted to hear more about cryoablation and asked the man if they could have a chat together after the group. I had no doubt that he would try to find a way of getting the man to face the need for further treatment without confronting him in public with what might be taken as a put-down.

I was at once envious and sorry—envious because this man had been spared incontinence and his sex life was unimpaired, sorry that in this case cryoablation was not the end of his problems, but possibly, unbeknownst to him, only the beginning.

The next man was a salesman, youngish, perhaps in his late thirties, but his body was bloated—not *fat*, as if he were an overeater, but *puffy*. His thighs strained the material of his trousers—he clearly had not yet bought new clothes—his shirt gaped open between the buttons, his suit jacket looked as if it were about to burst. His skin, now that I looked more closely, had an unhealthy pale yellowish tinge to it.

He had chosen hormone therapy over a radical prostatectomy, he said, and was happy with the result. His PSA was way down, and he was leading a perfectly normal life—about to get married, in fact.

I was impressed, but I could tell that the old hands were skeptical. The downside came quickly. He wanted to get off the hormones now that he was going to marry, because on them he had no sex drive. Hormone therapy, as I remembered from my talk with the radiologist at Memorial Sloan-Kettering, was chemical castration, a kinder, gentler (and less permanent) way of cutting off the body's ability to produce testosterone than the surgical removal of the testes. So long as the young man was willing to accept the loss of libido (and the physical changes), his cancer was more or less under control, although it was still *there,* an alien and malignant force held tenuously at bay by chemicals. The moment he stopped taking the hormones, the cancer would be released, ready to grow and multiply again. Like every prostate-cancer patient—I tried not to even *think* the word *victim*—he was faced with Hobson's choice: you couldn't halt the cancer without giving up something, in this case libido and potency.

Dennis gave the salesman the name of a couple of surgeons in the area he might want to consult, and a radiologist. He warned him that there was no easy solution: once you were on hormones, you couldn't just go off them like that, just because you were getting married.

I could see that the salesman was disappointed—as well he might be. This was a perfect example of somebody's *not* getting the kind of information he needed before making a decision, just the kind of thing that Dennis had been talking about.

A middle-aged, well-dressed man, a businessman, rose next. He felt some embarrassment, he said. He hadn't had any treatment at all—in fact, he had only just been told that he had cancer. An elevated PSA at his annual physical had led him to have a biopsy performed, and it had proved positive. "I'm hearing this, I'm hearing that," he said, "but what I want to know is: What should I do?"

"You've come to the right place," Dennis said. "What should he do?"

One by one, around the table, the regulars spoke up. One man—probably in his late seventies—put his hand up. "Listen to this guy," several people said. "*He* knows."

What we heard was a mixed story. The good news was that he was still alive fifteen years after having been diagnosed with prostate cancer. He had seen his grandchildren grow up; he and his wife still enjoyed life—these were good things, and he was grateful for them, no doubt about that. The bad news was that all along the way doctors had never told him the truth. He had a radical prostatectomy first, then, when the cancer reappeared, radiation, the aftereffects of which had been no fun. Maybe it was nobody's fault, maybe it was just one of those things, he wasn't blaming, but the radiation damaged his colon, so they had to give him a temporary colostomy, and ever since then he had a problem controlling his bowels, and if you thought *urinary* incontinence was bad, sonny—a glance in my direction— you should try *bowel* incontinence. Several people around the table sighed and nodded. One of them said, loudly, "Oy veh."

After that, the older man went on, he was on hormones for a long time, but the cancer kept coming on, eventually metastasizing to the bone. . . . So now he was on strontium 89 injections, one every two months, thousands of dollars apiece—can you believe it? Nobody in *this* audience found that hard to believe. I sensed that they had heard this story before, that it was something of a ritual, as much for the benefit of newcomers as anything else.

The speaker leaned his elbows against the table. He was neatly dressed in sporty resort clothes, as if he were on his way to play golf in Florida. "I will tell you this," he said, his voice dropping. "If I had it to do all over again, I would have taken five *good* years instead of the fifteen I've had. Five years of living like a real human being, able to make love, not having to worry about shitting in my pants, not going back for this treatment or that treatment, always with some side effect they didn't tell you about. . . . Somebody should have told me, is what I'm saying. Somebody should have warned me. Because if somebody had, I would have chosen differently, that's all. I would have taken the five years, lived them to the fullest, then taken what was coming and good-bye. Every day I think about it, and I wish I had, that's all I got to say."

The businessman—who was about fifty—looked stunned, as I would have been had I heard this before going down to Johns Hopkins. As others spoke up at the table, their stories, too, were a litany of decisions they felt they had been rushed into, without adequate explanation about the probable aftereffects.

There were exceptions—a middle-aged man who was a laborer with a construction company (and who had been operated on at Johns Hopkins, though not by Dr. Walsh) and me, as well as a few others—but most of the men around the table burned with resentment, once somebody had opened the floodgates.

"He said, 'Well, it's cancer, but I'm going to fix you up,' " one man told us, speaking of his urologist. "All he wanted to know was whether my insurance covered it. He didn't tell me, 'You might end up incontinent and impotent, and you might still have the cancer, even after all that.' If he'd told me that, believe me, I'd have thought it over. My wife is a very attractive woman, younger than me. This shouldn't have happened to her. It shouldn't have happened to me. We should have been warned."

I spoke up. I *was* warned, I said. Repeatedly, even in writing. Admittedly, the fear of cancer makes it hard to hear those warnings, and certainly once one has decided to opt for the surgery, the mind goes deaf to them—has to, I supposed, if only to avoid agonizing second thoughts—still, I couldn't say that I hadn't been warned.

There was some muttering at this, from which I took it that in many cases the warning had been perfunctory, or, in others, that the patient simply wasn't listening, perhaps out of fear, perhaps because some men, particularly those in blue-collar jobs, view their doctor as an authority figure—perhaps *the* authority figure—so when told that they have to have an operation, they fall meekly into line. The more educated the patient, I concluded, the more likely he was to ask questions and insist on a second opinion. Once they had survived whatever the first step was in their therapy, however, *all* the men in the room learned to ask questions.

Gently but firmly, Dennis brought the meeting back to order. You can see how hard it is to know what to do, he said to the man who had just been diagnosed with prostate cancer. A lot of people here would love to go back in time and do it a different way. Watchful waiting might work for you, maybe hormone treatments. Sure, the smart money is on a radical prostatectomy, maybe followed by hormones, but don't be rushed into anything, or proceed without a second opinion. In most cases, there is time.

I raised my hand. At Memorial, I said, they had an experimental program in which they put the patient on hormone therapy for six months, after which they performed a radical prostatectomy. They claimed that the hormones shrank the tumor and therefore lessened the chances of incontinence and impotence, since there was less tissue to remove.

Dennis nodded. That was the most important thing, he said approvingly. You had to keep looking for the experimental programs that your doctor probably *didn't* know about. Something new was being developed all the time, and we had to keep ourselves informed. Drug companies were trying out new medications, and it was sometimes possible to put yourself forward for the *in vivo* testing. You owed it to yourself to learn everything, and never, ever, to give up.

With that, it was nine P.M., and the meeting was over. Several people asked to know more about my condom catheter. The construction worker wanted to know how much Dr. Walsh had charged me for the operation, so he could tell whether his union had been overcharged. An elderly man told me not to lose hope. He had been incontinent for over a year, then one day, out of the blue, it had stopped, and he'd been dry ever since. The man who was on hormone therapy asked me for the name of a good book he could read about treatment for prostate cancer, and I suggested Dr. Rous's. I stirred Emory, who had been rocking back and forth on his chair near the door. What had he made of it? I asked. "It was a lot livelier than I thought it was going to be," he said. "I stayed awake for quite a bit of it."

THE EVENING HADN'T depressed me, as Dr. Josephy had feared it might. On the contrary, it had cheered me up, not so much because I had been exposed to men so much worse off than myself, but because even for the oldest and most afflicted of them there was (or had been at some point) hope. However crotchety they might be on the subject of the medical establishment, however much they might regret the choices that they had made, or that in certain cases had been forced on them, they were still alive, kicking, and complaining.

What mattered was to listen, learn, talk. What women do naturally, men have to learn, and for that reason alone the prostate-cancer survivors' group was a huge step in the right direction. If only these men had talked this way to one another *before* their surgeries, I told myself, half their misery would never have happened. Women talked about breast cancer with friends, with their families, with total strangers, and read about it in every magazine and newspaper. Those who were smart were as well-informed on the subject as many doctors were, maybe better. But in most cases, men didn't start learning about prostate cancer until they had it. Dennis was right; you simply couldn't have too much information. Even in my own case, I could already see that in some respects my fate *was* now in my own hands, like it or not. Dr. Walsh had given me the best operation he could—probably the best operation *anybody* could—but future choices and decisions I would have to make on my own—if there was, as they say, a sequel to my case—and I was more likely to pick up the latest scuttlebutt on prostate cancer here than anyplace else. And, anyway, where else could you talk about it man-to-man?

23

THE NEXT TIME I WENT BACK TO THE GROUP, I DROVE MYSELF (though still accompanied by Emory, just to be on the safe side). It was a huge leap forward, eight weeks after surgery, exactly on Dr. Walsh's schedule.

My voice was also beginning to return to its normal pitch, though I had not yet lost the breathlessness. My interest in work had returned, and telephone calls, manuscripts, and faxes were beginning to flood in—firmly controlled, however, by Margaret.

Somewhere along the way, I had apparently lost (or perhaps temporarily mislaid) the capacity to unravel complicated problems or sort out conflicting points of view. It was as if I had only so much energy to direct at a given subject, and when it was gone I didn't want to hear anything more about it—not the right frame of mind for somebody who prides himself on his negotiating skills and persuasiveness. I could actually *hear* myself getting snappy, but there was nothing I could do to stop it when it happened, as if I were listening to another—and far more querulous—person. I remembered what Larry McMurtry had written after his quadruple bypass:

> All that soon came to feel as if it belonged in another person's biography: the biography, for instance, of the person I had been before the operation. But I had ceased to be that person; I acted him or impersonated him as best I could, for the benefit of loved ones; I managed to retain certain of his abilities, but not all. . . .
>
> I have felt largely posthumous since the operation. My old psyche, or old self, was shattered—now it whirls around

me in fragments. I can generally gather enough of the fragments to make a fair showing, professionally and, I hope,
emotionally. But I am always conscious of working with
fragments of a self, never the whole.*

Of course, there is a world of difference between a quadruple bypass, in which the heart itself is stopped, and a radical prostatectomy,
but perhaps the consequences of all major surgery are alike—one returns from unconsciousness with deeper scars than the ones on the
surface, scars which, unlike the surface ones, don't ever heal completely.

Before, I had been able to push myself relentlessly. Now, I knew,
even though it was still the early days on the way to full recuperation,
that I would never feel the same about work again. Henceforth, I
would do what I *could,* and stop there. If people didn't like it, the hell
with them. I no longer wanted, really, to please anybody but myself,
something of a sea change for a person who had been working
twenty-four hours a day to please other people for most of his adult
life.

In the meantime, I concluded that Margaret was right. I needed to
stop working *before* I was tired, not wait until fatigue had already hit
me. Once that simple fact had sunk in, it was easier to deal with
things. "I'm sorry, but I need to rest now," I told people when I could
feel my body pulling me away from whatever problem my mind was
trying to grapple with. The person I *was* would never have said that.
The person I had become was perfectly at ease with it—and why not,
at the age of sixty-one?

At first I found the idea of having limited energy (and worse, a limited attention span) hard to accept, but then, very gradually, I was
able to put it in perspective. In the first place, I told myself, I was only
a few weeks away from major surgery; in the second place, I was recuperating from cancer. Either of these, let alone both, would be suf-
ficient to explain certain limitations on my activity. More important

* Printed by kind permission of Larry McMurtry.

was the realization—much delayed, some would say—that I was neither immortal nor young. Of course, in contemporary American society, sixty-one *isn't* exactly *old,* as we are forever being told. Like a lot
of sixty-year-olds, I exercised, dieted, kept fit and trim. I hardly felt
middle-aged, let alone old!

Of course, I was lucky, but then so are increasing numbers of
Americans who are making it into their sixties at the peak of their
earning ability, sexually active, still playing power tennis or whatever
their game is, probably in better shape than they were at forty, so free
of aches and pains that sixty-something merely seems like a way station to an immortality of melatonin, health spas, second or third
marriages, and new careers.

But cancer is a harsher teacher than inspirational bestsellers or ads
for vitamin-mineral supplements. It reminds us that we are *not* immortal, that our time is limited, that disease and death are still out
there waiting for us, unappeased by visits to the Golden Door, low-
fat diets, or a perky, upbeat attitude; that to be sixty-plus is, to put it
bluntly, no longer middle-aged but rather the first step toward old
age. *"Et in Arcadia Ego."* Cancer is the worm in the apple of jaunty
optimism about life; the banana peel on which even the healthiest
and fittest of us slips; a great teacher, if you're lucky enough to survive the lesson. Prostate cancer, by and large, is a disease that strikes
those in their sixties and over. For men in that age category, it
sounds—or *ought* to sound—a loud alarm. The way ahead is
marked, for prostate-cancer survivors, in clearly marked segments of
time, labeled "five-year survival," "ten-year survival," and "beyond."
Nobody who has had prostate cancer is going to think of himself as
immortal, not ever again, and it is a measure of our innocence that
those of us who have been lucky until then find that hard to accept.

Lying on my study sofa, trying to cope with the problems of incontinence, it began to dawn on me that age is an honorable state,
not to be lightly dismissed by pretending that one is eternally young,
or, worse still, eternally in midlife crisis. As a nation, we have begun
pretending that age doesn't really *exist,* that it's only a state of mind,

but that's like sitting at a play and pretending there's no second act, or that it won't be followed by the curtain. This has resulted in a certain dislike of the old, who, by simply being there, around us every day with their problems, put the lie to these illusions—which no doubt largely explains the meanspirited tone of recent political arguments about cutting Social Security, Medicare, and pensions. "Who *are* these old people who need more medical care and develop all sorts of physical problems, and why aren't they like the tanned, smiling, silver-haired, clear-eyed oldsters in the Geritol ads?" politicians and social thinkers seem to be asking. "Why aren't they out there becoming late-blooming entrepreneurs, or taking world cruises, or going back to college?" It's as if the whole country has decided that the old are malingerers, special pleaders stubbornly protecting too big a slice of the national economy, selfish for living too long. Age, in short, has become an unpopular notion, as people dedicate themselves more and more to the ideal of being forever young.

But age is real, and it's *different* from the earlier stages of life, not just an extension of middle age in which you move to Florida, or start getting Social Security checks. After all, a man of sixty-one is no longer a kid—if he feels like taking a nap, why shouldn't he? Perhaps it took cancer to get me to accept my age, to become *comfortable* with the idea of being—to call a spade a spade—*old,* but it's no small accomplishment in a culture that either ignores the fact or pretends that it's an unmitigated blessing.

Perhaps I had felt immortal before; I no longer did, nor did my fellow members of the prostate-cancer group—for, at my second meeting, I saw them more clearly. *"Mon semblable, mon frère,"* these angry, confused, and—let us be frank—*elderly* men were close to me in ways that those who had never gone through cancer could ever be.

—∾—

THE SECOND MEETING I went to was less confessional, partly because it was a "Two by Two" occasion, with wives invited. This time, there was a guest speaker—a young man from a blood-test laboratory who lectured us on PSA tests, giving us the news that the normal PSA test we were all accustomed to was not nearly sensitive enough for people who had undergone a radical prostatectomy, and that far more accurate tests were becoming available *if only doctors would specify them.*

Until then I had presumed—as do most physicians—that a PSA test is a PSA test, but this turned out not to be the case. PSA is usually measured in relatively broad strokes, which doesn't matter much because for most men the only questions worth asking are (1) is it over 4, and (2) has it gone up in the six months or a year since the last test? Once you have had a radical prostatectomy, however, the PSA should drop close to 0. If the operation is a complete success, the PSA may, in fact, be as low as 0.1 or less, which is fine, except that it *is,* as it turns out, possible to measure the PSA far more precisely than this, and thus monitor the most minute changes, rather than waiting until the PSA takes a significant leap upward.*

The lecturer was not exactly thrilling, even on a subject that was dear to his—or his company's—heart, but he nevertheless held the attention of this audience. Some were busily writing down significant facts about PSA; others, eyes half closed, crouched forward so as not to miss the one item of information, buried in all these statistics, that might apply specifically to their cases.

There was a certain religious quality, however improbable, to the meeting. The act of faith here was a stubborn belief in science, conventional or otherwise, the conviction that someone, somewhere,

---

* This new and more exact method of measuring and interpreting PSA is also of special interest as an *early* detector of prostate cancer. In the August 1995 *Journal of Urology,* Professor Joseph E. Oesterling, urologist-in-chief of Michigan Medical Center, Ann Arbor, drew the attention of physicians to look at "the ratio between two groups of molecules found in PSA, rather than at the total PSA level." Quoted in a news story in the *Milwaukee Journal Sentinel,* August 21, 1995, Dr. Oesterling explained that PSA is composed of "free" and "complexed" molecules, "the latter being associated with the presence of cancer." Urologists, Oesterling argues, should examine a patient's *molecular ratio* before performing a biopsy. The greater the ratio, the less the need for a biopsy. "With these new findings, a large number of patients can now avoid having a prostate biopsy without the risk of having a cancer missed," Dr. Oesterling commented. Clearly, the ability to detect the presence of prostate cancer without a biopsy, and to monitor the cancer's rate of growth, will bring about significant changes in the management of prostate cancer once this new test comes into widespread use.

had the answer to whatever one's problem was. The dullness of the lecture did not matter—it was a kind of penance, like listening to a tedious sermon. Perhaps, indeed, the duller and the more impenetrable, the better—for these people were worshiping at the shrine of medical science, searching for cures that, they believed, their doctors were ignorant of or, worse, were withholding. I did not envy the lot of their doctors when these men arrived with their notebooks full of newly won information.

Many people shared their numbers with the lecturer, including a man whose PSA had dropped from 80 to 30 in just over a year—entirely, he believed, because of his diet, which had also brought his cholesterol count down from 280 to under 200. Some of the men in this room, I reflected, had awesomely high PSA numbers and were yet still alive. I wondered what mine was, and what I would do if it were high. Everyone agreed that the first PSA test after surgery was critical. Even a small number, anything significantly above 0, in fact—unlikely though Dr. Walsh felt that was—would indicate the presence of cancer, despite the surgery that was intended to have removed it. I would have my first PSA test about twelve weeks after surgery. Until then, despite Dr. Walsh's satisfaction with the surgery he had performed, I was on probation.

The idea did not haunt me, although it oppressed Margaret, who felt that our lives would henceforth always be lived under the gun. And my answer then, as now, was yes, that's the way our lives *will* be lived, but why dwell on it? Everybody's life is measured out by the Fates, as the ancient Greeks knew, and they cut the skein with their shears when they choose to.

At the end of the meeting, Dennis repeated the themes of the evening: make *sure* your doctor prescribes the right PSA test for you, and don't take no for an answer.

"It's your life," he said, fastening his briefcase with a snap. "Not your doctor's." He paused as we stood up and milled around. "Never forget it," he added.

24

LUCKILY FOR ME, MY FIRST PSA TEST AFTER SURGERY WAS SOMETHING to celebrate. My number had dropped to 0.5, close to 0. I called Dr. Walsh, who was modestly pleased that his prediction had come true. Did I have any problems? I did my incontinence number while he listened patiently. I should not be concerned, he said. These things take time. I should see how things were going after six months. In the meantime, had I had any erections? I had not. Dr. Walsh was not dismayed. That would take time, too, he said. Perhaps a year. Perhaps more. I should be patient. The main thing was that my cancer was gone. I should call him again in two months' time.

I gave Ned a call to ask how *he* was doing. He was back at work, it seemed, and doing fine. Dr. Walsh had been pleased with his operation, too. And incontinence? I asked. Ned sighed. It was still pretty bad, he said. He was going through about six Depends a day—about the same number I was—in fact, he wished now that he'd had the foresight to buy shares in the company. And sex? A longer sigh. Nothing yet, he said, but what really depressed him was that Bob, who had waltzed through surgery with such little trouble, said that *his* sex life was back to "normal." That depressed me, too, until Ned added that he didn't think it was true.

As it turned out, it wasn't. Bob had been joking, it seemed—a joke no doubt somewhat tinged with bitterness, for of the three of us who had been operated on the same day, he was by far the most optimistic and self-confident.

The truth was that very few men escaped unscathed from a radical prostatectomy in some way. The numbers did not lie. *Eventually* the majority of men recovered some degree of potency (*if* they had possessed it before, *if* the nerve bundles were spared, *if* there were no other complications, like diabetes, etc.), but *eventually,* in the circumstances, was an elastic and imprecise word, not offering much in the way of comfort.

For the moment, however, potency was less an issue for me than incontinence.

—⁓—

SOME NOTION OF just how widespread incontinence is can be gleaned by the number and variety of people (and organizations) who claim to be able to help. Within a fairly short period of time I had consulted with a nutritionist, a yoga teacher, and several experts in biofeedback, and also joined an organization called HIP (Help for Incontinent People), with a newsletter (*The HIP Report*) dedicated to "Promoting Quality Continence Care" and an 800 number (1-800-BLADDER). Clearly, I had plenty of company.

My investigation of nutrition proved only moderately helpful, though it is very likely that any prostate-cancer patient will benefit to some degree from taking the right mix of vitamins and minerals. This is a subject doctors don't take much if any interest in. I was prescribed iron pills *prior* to my surgery, to avoid anemia while I was giving blood, but nobody paid the slightest attention to that *after* my surgery, with the result that I did, in fact, develop anemia, by no means uncommon in surgical patients who have experienced blood loss—not a serious problem, but an avoidable one, which might never have been discovered if I hadn't complained constantly of fatigue. A consultation with a nutritionist is probably a good idea for anybody who has had surgery, even if it doesn't offer an instant cure for incontinence.

Yoga, I found, has plenty of exercises designed to strengthen the muscles of the pelvic region. Further, it's a way of toning the muscles *without* the heavy lifting and the physical exertion that a patient recovering from abdominal surgery ought to avoid, and it offers an effective, long-term way of helping the body to recover. Calmness has an effect on incontinence, in fact. When the mind is calm and un-troubled, the urge to urinate tends to diminish; when the mind is upset and distracted, the urge is far more powerful and frequent.

Neither nutrition nor yoga should be ignored, I decided, and I in-corporated both into my daily regime, with some success. Biofeed-back sounded more exciting, perhaps because it is "Western" and "scientific." A researcher in the psychology department at Columbia-Presbyterian Hospital, in New York City, admitted that biofeedback *was* being used effectively in cases of female incontinence, particu-larly after childbirth. So far as he knew, both the software and the hardware were intended for women, not men (the equipment he was referring to is, in fact, called the Vagette, and was designed for the electrostimulation of the female urinary tract), but he gave me the names of several doctors, one of whom finally put me in touch with Dr. Howard Glazer, who was *the* expert in biofeedback for male in-continence, and surprisingly helpful.

Yes, Dr. Glazer said, biofeedback *did* work very well for male in-continence, and he had had a very high rate of success among pa-tients who had undergone a radical prostatectomy. The procedure was straightforward, but neither cheap nor instantaneous, the major inconvenience being that I would need to order the necessary equip-ment first, before I could begin with the treatment. I would need an anal EMG sensor and a portable EMG "home trainer" unit. The idea, as he described it, involved placing the anal sensor, which was attached by wires to the EMG unit, in the rectum. It was then possi-ble to isolate exactly the muscle groups that needed to be exercised and carry out these exercises specifically. In short, while most men doing Kegel exercises couldn't be sure that they were doing them ef-fectively, by means of biofeedback you could ensure that you were reaching *exactly* the right muscles and exercising them correctly, and you could actually *measure* progress scientifically, instead of relying on the vague notion that you did the exercises until you got tired.

This was the good news. The bad news was that Dr. Glazer didn't feel it was worth doing any of this until I had given myself at least six months, or even a year, to recover continence by myself. "It's too early," he said. "Do the Kegel exercises, and call me back in three months." He dismissed both Dr. Walsh's prohibition against doing Kegel exercises and the usual recommendation of doing a half a dozen of them two or three times a day. *His* patients did them by the *hundreds,* in series, and the relaxation between each contraction, I should remember, was as critical as the contraction. He was doubtful, he added, that a patient could do himself any good by doing exercises *without* biofeedback, although his feeling was, unlike Dr. Walsh, that he probably couldn't do himself any great harm, either.

The HIP newsletter, when it finally arrived, was initially something of a disappointment. It turned out to be basically an advertising gimmick supported by manufacturers of incontinence products, among them Attends briefs, the Tranquillity Pad and Pant system, the Secure system of bedside drainage, and Nullo internal deodorant tablets. There is, of course, no reason why manufacturers of such products shouldn't fund a newsletter, and there was quite a lot of useful information in it, but the tie-in made me wary. On the other hand, had I not read the HIP newsletter, I would have remained unaware that certain medications can bring on incontinence (or that there exists a twenty-four-hour-a-day hot line to check your prescription for just such problems) or that the female workers of Nabisco had filed a federal sex-discrimination suit because the company didn't allow enough bathroom breaks. I was clearly not the only person in America for whom the ease of access to a bathroom loomed large as a concern.

Reading *The HIP Report* also gave me a comforting feeling, both because there were a lot of people out there worse off than myself (a *lot* worse off), and because there were plenty of organizations designed to help people cope with the problem, not to speak of a long reading list.

When it came to Kegel exercises, HIP, I noted, took the view that ten contractions three times a day for men recuperating from a radical prostatectomy were ample,* and had available both a cassette tape and a leaflet on how to perform them correctly. Both, when they arrived, were helpful, clear, and contradicted both Dr. Walsh and Dr. Glazer.

—⁂—

BY THIS TIME, more than twelve weeks since the surgery, I was ready to go back to the office. I limited my first day to two hours, in the morning, then I went back to our city apartment, had a light lunch, and took a rest.

This proved to be about as much as I could take at the beginning. I avoided lunch dates altogether, as well as long meetings, so as not to have to sit too long—prolonged sitting was still a misery. I filled my briefcase with extra Depends, and confronted, for the first time, the slight embarrassment of having to change and dispose of them in a public bathroom. In the end, I coped, as everybody copes. As handicaps go, incontinence, I discovered, is comparatively minor. The only person who is likely to be aware of the problem is oneself. It can be lived with.

What was harder to live with, oddly enough, was the simple strain of being in the city itself. I walked the few blocks from the apartment to the office in a state of real physical fear, terrified of people, of traffic, of everything. There was also another fear: that somehow my incontinence would be obvious to people. Peculiar to fear this, Margaret said, considering my tendency to talk too much about it, to bring people's attention to it when there was no need to. It is an occupational hazard of cancer, whatever form it takes, this need to talk about it.

Still, there *were* improvements. My scar was fading, and with it, many of my postsurgical symptoms. I was dry enough at night to give up my Depends in bed for a pair of Sir Dignity briefs, which looked for all the world like ordinary Jockey shorts, except for a discreet plastic pouch in front, where the fly would normally be, into

---

* DeLancey, J. O.; Sampselle, C. M.; and Punch, M. R.; *Obstet Gynecol 1993;* 82:658–659, as quoted in *The HIP Report,* vol. 13, no. 12.

which a replaceable absorbent pad fitted. Sir Dignity briefs *looked* like normal underwear, and felt normal, too.

At first, I wasn't too sure of them, but I soon discovered that they worked just fine, and before long I was able to get through the night on just one pad. I was not ready yet to wear them during the day, while I was exercising or walking around, and not confident enough to wear them while I was driving or sitting in a car.

Before long, my confidence was such that the trappings of incontinence at home could be removed: the mattress pad, the mats on the floor, the pads on the sofa and on the car seat. The urinals I kept, just to be on the safe side, and they proved worthwhile, for on one trip down to the city, with Margaret driving me, I was saved from disaster by being able to piss into the urinal, with the car pulled over on the side of the road.

The problem was still the unpredictable urgency and frequency of urination, very much worse than it had ever been before surgery. I could put it in perspective now: a misfortune, a mild handicap with occasional moments of humiliation, but a lot better than, say, cancer in the lymph nodes or metastasized to the bone. Sometimes, very rarely, my urinary problems would drive me into a fit of anger at my inability to control this most basic of functions, but on the whole I was managing to get on with my life.

SOON MY WORKING day expanded from two hours to four, to six, then, before long, to something approaching normal. I was having lunch dates again—eating in a restaurant, like a civilized person—skipping my afternoon nap, running (rather tentatively) instead of taking a walk, in short, resuming my normal, presurgery, life.

Sometimes I had doubts about just that, which Margaret and I discussed often and at length. While I was recuperating, lying on my back, legs up, it had seemed to me that our life should somehow be *different* after the ordeal, or what was the point? Like every patient I daydreamed: I would take early retirement, we would cruise down the Nile, I would spend more time, perhaps *all* my time, in the country—"Nobody on his deathbed ever wishes he'd spent more time in the office."*

True enough, but as my strength returned, perhaps the most important discovery I made was that I *liked* my life, that I *needed* my work. I could not control the return of continence or sexual potency (or even, though I tried not to think about it, the return of my cancer), but I *could* control my work—here, at least, was an area in which I had potency, and at least for a time it would have to offset the rest.

Not that I didn't make some changes, overdue for a man of sixty-one, going on sixty-two as I write this. I learned to take a rest when I needed it, I stopped getting up at dawn to work, I made a valiant effort to end the working day by five, replaced—as Margaret pointed out—an obsessive compulsion to work with an obsessive compulsion to exercise. I also found, perhaps for the first time in my life, a certain kind of peace, a protection, thin and fragile, but still there, against all the normal, everyday angst, stress, and problems of my work. Things might go wrong—surely would do so—but nothing that was likely to happen at work could be as bad as hearing that you have cancer, or living through whatever procedures were necessary to overcome it and survive. If nothing else, cancer puts the everyday troubles of the working day in perspective.

—∿—

FIVE MONTHS AFTER my surgery, going on six, my recuperation seemed complete. I was back to my usual schedule, working on this book, writing a piece for *The New Yorker*, driving myself to and from the city, beginning to look, as people told me constantly, like my old self again (though the face I saw in the mirror was still that of a stranger); *recovered*, they said.

* Oddly, this quote is widely attributed to Vincent Foster, the counsel to the president who committed suicide in July 1993.

PART FOUR

RECOVERY

25 Today

Successful recuperation is when your friends and your doctors think you're doing well, and back to normal again; recovery is when *you* think you've arrived there, physically *and* mentally. There's a big difference.

By that standard, I still have a long way to go, nine months after surgery as I write this. With my PSA down to 0.1, about as low as it can get, my cancer is behind me, just as Dr. Walsh had promised it would be, and I am duly grateful for the fact. The rest I am learning to take one day at a time, without becoming discouraged, just as Dr. Walsh advised.

Really, when I think back on it, I got off lightly. Nine months of disruption, discomfort, and fear, followed by what has been so far (touch wood!) a clean bill of health—I'm a lucky man, compared to friends who, in the same period of time, have undergone bone-marrow transplants, or had a lung removed, followed by chemotherapy, or been diagnosed with cancer of the stomach that has spread to the bile duct. . . . Every time I hear about things like that, I thank my lucky stars.

There's a mystery to cancer, far beyond the medical or biological facts of the disease. Somehow this body—not only "mine," but *me*—developed, through no fault of my own that I can imagine, an organism determined to kill me. It's hard to think of your own body as a battlefield, or your own DNA as a potential killer, but that's the fact. In cancer, the body becomes the enemy, attempting to destroy itself.

Against cancer, as against no other disease, we wage the equivalent of "total war." It's kill-or-be-killed time, we throw in everything we've got to destroy the enemy before the enemy destroys us, and during the process there's a certain exhilaration of the kind which invariably accompanies war, a powerful adrenaline rush that sees one through the worst of it.

With victory, there comes an inevitable reckoning of the cost, a counting of our losses. Yes, we have won (thank God!), but look at what we sacrificed to win, and was the sacrifice really necessary?

Such thoughts follow any victory in war (the losers have other problems to worry about). Was it worth it? people ask. If we had it to do all over again, would we have done the same thing?

Might I have been better off *not* having a radical prostatectomy, people ask me, considering what the effects of it have been on my life? I do my best to answer that kind of question, but really, like the questions historians ask about the past, what's the point? Even if I *could* go back in time again, cancer is cancer, and sitting around gambling that it's the "slow-growing" kind, like some men I have known who died from doing just that, seems plain *dumb*. Radiation wasn't deemed appropriate for me because my prostate was enlarged, nobody suggested hormone therapy, cryoablation remains a question mark, and that leaves surgery as the only approach.

I picked the best surgeon, at one of the finest medical institutions in the world, so I had no reproaches against myself or anybody else. Certainly, I could wish that I had gone to Memorial Sloan-Kettering for my biopsy when my PSA was first brought to my attention. I think it's possible—not *sure,* mind you, but possible—that I might have been diagnosed with prostate cancer a year or eighteen months earlier, and that might well have made the surgery far less difficult and spared me a good many of the consequences.

If men talked to one another about prostate cancer, I'd have been more aware of the importance of the PSA test, more concerned about what an elevated PSA might indicate, less inclined to leave well enough alone after the first biopsy. If I'd taught myself what I *now* know about prostate cancer *then,* I'd have asked more questions and insisted on answers. . . .

—◊◊◊—

BUT THEN THAT'S the lesson of this book: some 200,000 American men are going to find out that they have prostate cancer this year, and most of them don't have a clue what it involves, or what their choices are, or what they should know (or even what questions they should ask), and won't find out until it's too late.

A rule of thumb: if your wife knows more about breast cancer than *you* know about prostate cancer, then maybe there's something you should be learning from her, right now, since the statistics are about the same. Women's magazines are full of stories about cancer—women's health issues share equal billing with fashion and beauty in the world of women's magazines. Compare that to men's magazines, in which illness is never mentioned. Women pick up at least *some* of the information they need from what they read. Men pick up next to nothing.

Even the simplest kind of information would help—perhaps just repeating over and over again the importance of a PSA test, for example. Of course, keeping up with the latest findings in the field of prostate cancer isn't easy, even for those who have a good reason to do so. For one thing, things change rapidly in medicine. As we have seen, the new and more highly refined PSA tests, for example, will give doctors a way of determining just how malignant the tumor is, and what its rate of growth may be, thus making it perhaps unnecessary to perform surgery on men with small, slow-growing prostate tumors, and instead more reasonable to subject them to "watchful waiting." Perhaps, then, hormone therapy can hold back the slow-growing tumors sufficiently so that over a man's lifetime no other treatment may be called for, and the radical prostatectomy as "the gold standard" for prostate cancer will be a thing of the past, except in cases where the tumor is advanced and fast-growing. In the meantime, however, we are still left with Hobson's choice between a treatment that disrupts or may permanently alter life, and a disease which may end it.

Even as I write these words, a story in the local paper quotes (as if it were a breathless scientific scoop) a recent study as suggesting that "watchful waiting" may be the best treatment (or, rather, *nontreatment*) for men over sixty-five with prostate cancer—that statistically, they die at about the same age as men who *don't* have prostate cancer. But this, as we have seen, is not news, and indeed is already the norm in Europe and the United Kingdom. The problem with that approach, however, is that a number of men over the age of sixty-five with prostate cancer have relatively fast-growing tumors, and who in his right mind wants to sit around waiting to find that out (only to discover the fact when it's too late)?

We are not, as a nation, much attracted to the passive approach to anything, let alone cancer. Of course, if and when the more advanced test for PSA which I have mentioned above becomes current, things will, very likely, be different, but for the moment all "good news" about prostate cancer should probably be taken with a grain of salt.

It is still killing about 50,000 American men a year, most of whom need not have died when they did, let alone have suffered such an awful death.

—∾—

RECOVERY MEANS COMING to terms at last with what has happened to you, "putting it all behind you," as they say—the cancer, the surgery, and all the rest of it. Usually, you can fix a date when it happens. For me, it was about nine months after the operation, at the end of a beautiful summer day in the country, when I slipped into bed and realized that I hadn't thought about my operation or my cancer once during the whole day, that it no longer figured at all in my plans or my thoughts.

That is not to say that the aftereffects were gone, or forgotten, but I had come to terms with them for the moment, made my peace with life as it had been offered to me. My life, whatever its defects, was a lot better than no life at all.

At nine months, the incontinence problem has been reduced to a level I can live with, most of the time, bar the occasional accident. I'm not happy about it, but I'm not miserable, either. As to the future, I have a few decisions to make. Should I live with a degree of incontinence permanently, or do something about it? If the latter, then what?

Biofeedback remains a possibility—something to consider when a year is up. There is talk that certain patients benefit from collagen injections to fill up the space left by the removal of tissue during the prostatectomy, but collagen moves around, and besides, it's an invasive procedure. I haven't found anybody who's actually *had* such an injection, but it's on my list to inquire about. I'm not so badly off that I'd contemplate a surgical implantation—having to wear a pad, getting the occasional "spurt" of urine at moments of physical stress, needing to keep within a reasonable (and predictable) ETA of a bathroom; none of these is enough to make me contemplate further surgery.

My inclination is to stick with Dr. Walsh's opinion that it will get better and that there's always time to change my mind. In the meantime, I try not to think too much about what is a comparatively minor physical handicap. Most of the time, I succeed.

—⁂—

IT'S A LITTLE harder to be philosophical about sex. So far as Dr. Walsh is concerned, I'm right on schedule, and maybe he's right—he never promised me a rose garden. Sexual feeling has returned, just as he said it would, but I've had no erections to speak of, although an occasional, twitchy beginning of one, despite my having only one nerve bundle to operate on, gives me hope that Dr. Walsh is correct.

According to Dr. Walsh, I shouldn't anticipate anything more until a year to eighteen months after surgery, so he's not concerned. Dr. Josephy's view is more pessimistic, but then I'm not really any more anxious to have an implant for erectile dysfunction than one for incontinence. (You can't have *both,* by the way—there's a limit to how much plastic plumbing can be installed in a human being.)

On the off chance that my progress might be speeded up (or even jump-started), I paid a visit to Dr. J. Francois Eid, at the New York Hospital–Cornell Medical Center's Sexual Function Center, in New York City, the state-of-the-art facility for men's sexual problems, a building so modern, elegant, and tastefully furnished that it seemed unlikely that any of the baser human physical functions could be served there.

Considering the problems of Dr. Eid's patients, it seemed to me cruel, whether by design or by accident, that his nurses looked like beauty-contest winners, though on reflection, the intention may have been to encourage the patients to proceed with their treatment. In any event, there was certainly a startling contrast between the glum-looking men, mostly well-dressed and middle-aged, in the waiting room and the members of Dr. Eid's staff flashing past in their short white coats.

Eid himself was tall, youngish, athletic, and good-looking, with an almost imperceptible French accent and a cheerful "can do" attitude toward sexual function. He listened to my story sympathetically. The walls of the examination room I was in—there were several, the center is a kind of factory of male sexuality—bore elaborate posters advertising a pocket-size kit for self-injection, as well as for Dr. Eid's book, *Making Love Again.* Before I was finished telling him about my surgery he handed me a gown and asked me to strip.

As Dr. Eid examined me, he gave me the doomsday scenario which is at the core of his thesis: the more erectile dysfunction (he does not condone the use of the word *impotence*) continues, the more muscle tissue in the penis atrophies. The longer the patient puts off treatment, the less effective it will be, and the smaller the erection. He considers it such a severe problem that he recommends beginning a course of treatment as early as possible after surgery.

This came as news to me—*unwelcome* news, doubly so since it flatly contradicted Dr. Walsh's optimism (though Dr. Eid professed something approaching reverence for Walsh's surgical skill). I had assumed that I had all the time in the world to wait and see, but Dr. Eid was assuring me of the contrary. There were, he said, warming to his subject, basically three approaches. The first was the vacuum pump, either hand-operated or, in the more deluxe version, electric. This was a device by means of which the patient placed a transparent tube over his penis, secured it with an O-ring, then pumped the air out, producing a vacuum. The tube was removed, leaving the O-ring in place at the base of the penis, and an erection resulted. The erection would last for some time, at least half an hour, or as long as the O-ring was in place, and would be more than adequate for intercourse, though not necessarily as straight as a normal erection.

I nodded. I liked the sound of the vacuum pump; it was not invasive, and seemed like a modest technological step in the right direction, an *aid*, rather like a cane or a crutch, with which one could dispense later. This hope Dr. Eid dashed. He was not an uncritical fan of the vacuum pump, and he did not think it would work for me. Any degree of incontinence would be a problem, he explained, since the action of the pump would almost certainly draw urine into the machine.

His recommendation was self-injection. The good news was that the new drugs were far more effective than Papaverine, which had been popular among Hollywood sexual athletes in the 1970s, and which, in the wrong dose, had a tendency to produce priapism, an erection which would not subside until the user was injected with an antidote (in some cases, the patient might even need an emergency operation to solve the problem). Now, Dr. Eid said, a "cocktail," a mixture of drugs tailored exactly to one person's needs which would produce exactly the required erection without pain or aftereffects, could be fashioned for every patient. Mixing my particular cocktail would take some trial and error, but it was not a lengthy process. After that, all I had to do was to inject myself in the penis—*twice*, actually, once on each side—and shortly afterward I would have an erection. In an hour or so, perhaps a little less, it would subside, and that was that.

I tried to think about the number of times in my life I had had an erection lasting an hour. They were not numerous. Then I tried to imagine injecting myself twice in the penis before making love. I did not think I could do it, and said so.

Dr. Eid frowned. There was nothing to it. He pointed to the poster. I would have a neat little black leather pouch, my own mixture, and a patented, easy-to-use, virtually painless syringe with which to inject myself. His patients were enthusiastic about it. He had no doubt I would feel the same.

I wasn't sure it was for me at all, I said. Dr. Eid smiled. I would see shortly, he said. He could do nothing without first testing to see how much atrophy had set in. If I would lie back, please, he would proceed with the injection, and I would see how easy it was.

Maybe I was making a fuss over nothing, I told myself. Maybe the injections were the answer. Dr. Eid produced a syringe with a long, fine needle, and filled it. I shut my eyes. How much could it hurt, after all? Surely I had been through much worse.

I felt a sharp stab in the right side of my penis as Dr. Eid injected his cocktail into it. I clenched my fists, and gave out a cry. "You have to relax," he said. "It's no good if I don't get the needle in deep."

"Relax?"

"It won't work if you don't relax. Please unclench your fists."

I tried, but they might as well have been glued shut. My fingernails were digging deep into my flesh and my muscles were rigid. Besides, it wasn't just my *fists* that were clenched—*everything* in my body was clenched, except for my penis, which remained flaccid.

"Now the other side," he said.

My behavior as Dr. Eid injected the left side of my penis was craven enough to shake his very considerable sangfroid. I tried to imagine doing this to myself, and failed. After all, he was a doctor; he presumably *knew* how to give injections. Even if I practiced a lot on oranges, I did not think I could plunge the needle into my own penis myself. Still, many people *did*, I reminded myself.

I felt him withdraw it. "Good," he said. "You see? What did I tell you? It was nothing." He told me to stand up—the injection works best if the patient stands after it has been administered, and it may even be necessary for him to perform intercourse either standing or kneeling. He opened a drawer and handed me two issues of *Penthouse* and one of *Playboy.* I was to flick through these and arouse myself while I stood. He would return in fifteen minutes or so to observe the result. Moodily, I swayed from bare foot to bare foot, flicking through the photographs in the magazines, while my penis throbbed. Seldom, if ever, had pornography had less effect on me. Not even the *Penthouse* Pet of the Month (for July of the previous year, I noted with an editor's eye), fingering the folds of her vagina as she smiled wistfully toward the camera, could arouse anything in me except a deep desire to be somewhere else and an overwhelming sense of how ridiculous my position was. Still, I reminded myself, almost everything to do with sex *was* ridiculous, if you thought about it long enough.

I was interrupted in this train of thought by the arrival of the erection Dr. Eid had promised. It was not, perhaps, an erection on a scale to excite fans of XXX-rated movies, but it was definitely there. And it hurt like hell.

It occurred to me, standing there looking at *Playboy,* that most of my life women have been telling me that sex isn't *about* erections, or penetration, it is about feelings, love, communication, contact— words which fell on deaf ears, in my case, as they do in the case of practically all men. I will not say that there have been no moments in my life when I understood what they *meant* (without necessarily *be- lieving* them), but the advice played little or no part in my own feelings about sexual intercourse or male sexual identity. Erection and penetration seemed to me what it was about, although I was open to other activities if sufficiently persuaded. Now, suddenly, I got the picture. After all, here I was, with a perfectly good erection, without even the slightest trace of sexual desire, no matter how earnestly I studied *Playboy*'s Playmate for May 1995.

On a mechanistic level, yes, I was erect, but in no other way could I be said to be "aroused." If one of Dr. Eid's attractive nurses had entered the room and torn off her clothes, I would have asked her to put them back on again. My penis throbbed with pain, rather than desire, and I reached, belatedly, the sad conclusion that the women in my life had been more knowledgeable about sex than I was.

When Dr. Eid reappeared (by that time, since he was delayed, I was actually *reading* the sex magazines, as if they were *The New York Times,* rather than looking at the pictures of girls), the first thing I asked him, to his surprise (and mine), was just how soon the erection would subside.

"In another half an hour," he said, a bit miffed, I thought, by my lack of appreciation.

"It's just that it hurts. I won't need an antidote, will I?"

"Probably not. Give it a bit of time." Dr. Eid gloved himself and played with my semitumescent organ. "You shouldn't wait too long before treatment," he said.

I said that I wasn't sure I could hack the injections. My reaction to the ones he had given me was apparently vivid enough in Dr. Eid's mind to make him drop the subject for the moment. If I had trouble with the idea of injecting myself, he said, I might want to consider an implant. Earlier implant mechanisms had not been entirely satisfactory, but the new ones—and, if he said so himself, nobody in the whole world was better at putting them in than he himself—were a huge step ahead, medical technology in its finest form. The patient reaches down, presses on a pump imbedded surgically in his scrotum, and—*voilà!*—an erection that lasts for as long as he (or his partner) likes. Once sex is over, he merely presses again, and the penis detumesces. No danger of priapism, no painful side effects, no sudden middle-of-the-night visits to the emergency room—the whole thing is so discreet, effective, and up-to-date that the patient's partner need never even know about it.

He examined my penis critically. "You've already got a certain amount of atrophy," he said. "We need to do a further test to measure the blood flow to the penis."

"Does that involve another injection?"

Dr. Eid rolled his eyes. "Yes," he said firmly, not apparently in a mood to sugarcoat the pill this time. "But it has to be done. Make an appointment with my secretary, please."

He rose to leave, but I called him back. "You're *sure* it will go down?" I asked, feeling a little guilty—after all, the man had promised me an erection, I had one, and now all I wanted was to get rid of it—but the fact was that it still ached and, until it subsided, I couldn't get dressed.

"Fifteen minutes, half an hour. If it doesn't, tell the nurse when she comes for you."

In about twenty minutes, the erection had subsided.

The nurse arrived and, once I was dressed, conducted me into a small office where a television set waited for me, so I could watch a half-hour video on sex aids in which well-groomed men and women with blow-dried hair, mostly of a certain age, described their satisfaction with one or another of the devices Dr. Eid and I had discussed.

I felt curiously relieved and cheerful as I walked over to First Avenue and entered a coffee shop. There was a row of magazines on the wall. I discreetly averted my eyes from *Penthouse* and *Playboy*, and bought a copy of *The New York Times*—an anaphrodisiac if ever there was one. Over coffee and a bagel, I mulled over my experience. It had not left me downhearted—on the contrary, I felt a good deal of admiration for Dr. Eid. He had put to rest any fears I might have had about permanent impotence. If I chose to take advantage of them, the means existed to achieve an erection. Dr. Eid had agreed, albeit with some reluctance, that it would do no harm to at least *try* the vacuum pump, if only as a way of preventing further atrophy. Eventually, if the problem persisted, I could pursue one of his more permanent solutions. It was up to me.

Most important, I had the information I needed, and with it the sense of pressure diminished, along with the fear that I would never be able to have sex again. "Do not become discouraged!" Dr. Walsh had written, and I was not. If Walsh was right, then patience was necessary, and the ability to have an erection would return in its own good time. If he was wrong—or I lost patience—then at least I knew that Dr. Eid could help me, in any way I chose.

In the meantime, I was alive, and that was what mattered. The rest, I was convinced, would solve itself in time, and if it did not, then I would move on to the next stage and decide what I could live with and what I couldn't. Maybe I'd get used to the injections, if that was what I decided on; maybe once the incontinence was more under control, I'd be able to use the vacuum pump on a regular basis; if all else failed, there was always the implant. In any case, medical technology was moving forward rapidly, as Dr. Eid had explained to me. There was talk of patches (like those for giving up smoking) replacing the injections, or even of the medication being available in the form of an eyedropper, so all you had to do was drop x number of drops into the penis, then wait for an erection.

Whatever I did, I would know when it was time, and I would know, too, how far I wanted to go. And I would not decide without knowing exactly what Margaret's feelings on the subject were.

Every day since then has brought small improvements so far as sex is concerned; the ability to have orgasm has returned in small, slow stages and although as yet there are no real signs of erection returning, beyond a few hopeful twinges, my visit to Dr. Eid made me much more philosophical on the subject than I had ever been or expected to be. Yes, he is probably right about the problem of atrophy, but it may not be as crucial as he believes, and in any case, the important thing is to know that there's help out there when and if I decide it's needed. Knowing that, I can relax and let sex return at its own pace, as Dr. Walsh had said it would, just as continence has done. The body, as my yoga instructor keeps telling me, heals at its own pace, and can't be hurried.

None of it worries me anymore. It is as if cancer itself had inoculated me against lesser fears. I had learned, as AA regulars do, to live one day at a time and take what each day brings without worrying too much about the next one—and that is no small lesson to have learned.

IN THAT SENSE, more than nine months after surgery, I have "recovered"—not recovered what I had, or who I was, before the call from Kathy in Dr. Russo's office changed my life. I do not think that will ever happen, and perhaps I no longer care. I'm not sure I *liked* that person nearly as much as I do the one I am now, or that the life I had then was as good as I thought it was. No, recovery comes, in the end, from the dawning realization that cancer was an *episode* in one's life, neither the end of it nor, more important, the whole of it.

John Wayne once said that his proudest achievement was that he had "licked the Big C." Of course, he hadn't. The Big C came back, and licked him, in the end. Nobody is really a match for cancer, not even the Duke. I do not pride myself that I have licked cancer. I survived a match with it, that's all. With any luck, it won't come back for a rematch, but if it does, I won't be afraid. We are all going to die of *something*. Nobody gets out of here alive.

IN THE END, my experience with prostate cancer seems to me a hopeful, optimistic one, not so much because I appear to be doing well—though that's gratifying—but because it proves to me that cancer, this particular brand of it, anyway, *can* be overcome, that it doesn't *have* to be the scary experience, appearing unexpectedly out of the blue, that it was for me. The information is out there, reams of it; new discoveries are being made every day; there's no *mystery* about it. The important thing is to know everything you can about the disease, and I'm keeping up on it, from day to day, relying on friends who send me clippings of the latest news and advances, and above all on my prostate-cancer support group, to keep me up-to-date and informed. Nothing could have *prevented* my cancer—after all, nobody knows what caused it in the first place—but what a difference it would have made if I'd been as well-informed on the subject as I am now. It happened to me, and I was unprepared for it, totally ignorant.

It *can* happen to you, too. These days, when I meet a man, I'm as likely as not to ask him what his PSA is. If he doesn't know, I urge him to find out. I am still astonished—and appalled—by the number of men who *don't* know, or can't remember, or who haven't been told by their doctors.

There is no reason why 50,000 American men a year should die from sheer ignorance, or from turning a blind eye to a disease which is so easily diagnosed at an early stage. Quite simply, the best cure for prostate cancer is to know as much as you can about it *before* it happens to you.

Learning about it the hard way, after you've been diagnosed as having it, may be the biggest mistake you'll ever make.

26

THERE ARE SIMPLE RULES FOR SURVIVING PROSTATE CANCER.

1. Have your PSA taken every year, and know what it is.
2. If it goes into the "danger area," or shows signs of rising steadily, have your biopsy done at the very best clinical facility you can find in your area, preferably at a hospital with a first-rate urology department. Talk to your doctor frankly about this. You have the right to the best possible biopsy, and your life may depend on it.

Above all, insist upon seeing the results and having them explained to you until you understand them. Don't be afraid of appearing ignorant or asking dumb questions. Don't be afraid that the doctor may think you're a pain in the ass. Your life is more important than what your doctor happens to think about you, and it's part of his job to explain things to you so that you understand *exactly* what your results mean.

3. If you are diagnosed as having prostate cancer, seek out *at least* a couple of other opinions from doctors not affiliated with yours. Do not decide on a course of treatment without at least one second opinion. Do not hesitate to ask around for the best urologist in your area, or to consult a book like *The Best Doctors in America*** for the name of the best-qualified urologist within reach. Most important, *inform yourself.* Read everything you can (at least the books I have mentioned), go to your local American Cancer Society and find out if they have a prostate-cancer group and attend a few meetings, talk to the men there, and seek out men who have had prostate cancer and talk to *them.* They will be familiar with most of the treatments that your doctor may propose to you, and perhaps more familiar than he is with the consequences of them. They may also have strong opinions about a given urologist or hospital. Listen to them. They have been there. Above all, remember that your life and your well-being depend on the informed choices *you* make. Your doctor can *present* you with those choices (and ought to do so objectively, and in layman's terms), but he cannot *decide* for you, nor should you expect him to.

4. Above all, do not panic. The more you know, the more likely you are to do well, both in the short run and in the long run. Your knowledge of the disease—and of your own case—as well as your will to survive, are what you have going for you.

---

* A reference work by Steven Naifeh and Gregory White Smith, published by Woodward/White in Aiken, South Carolina; latest edition: 1994–95.

5. If you're taking the surgery route, do not choose a surgeon until you have studied his credentials, his numbers (which should be compared with those of other surgeons), and talked to him frankly about your fears and questions. If you don't like him, or he won't discuss his numbers, see somebody else. This is not the time to be polite or to succumb to your doctor's idea of what constitutes good patient behavior. You have to have confidence in your surgeon, both on a personal level and by having ascertained that he is fully qualified and has performed (successfully) a large number of similar operations. Do not be overawed. Surgery is a job, like any other, and it's up to him to convince you he's the right man for you.

6. Be patient. It's a long haul, with many ups and downs. You need your strength, and you need as much support from family, friends, and loved ones as you can get. Peace of mind matters, so take your time and get the rest of your life in order before embarking on treatment.

7. If you decide in favor of a radical prostatectomy, anticipate a long recuperation, and make plans for it.

8. Remember: most prostate-cancer patients who receive treatment early enough live out a full actuarial life span. The numbers are on your side.

9. Don't suffer alone. Go find somebody who has the same problem and talk to him. He'll feel better; so will you.

10. Above all, never, ever give up hope.

APPENDIX

Helping Hands

Man to Man is an account of my own personal experience with prostate cancer, not a complete guide to the subject in the formal sense. For more detailed and prescriptive information I advise the reader to consult *The Prostate Book* by Dr. Rous, which I mention several times in the course of my narrative, and perhaps also Dr. Patrick C. Walsh's book *The Prostate* (Johns Hopkins Press). Numerous publications are also available from your local chapter of the American Cancer Society.

A short list follows of other resources that may be helpful to prostate cancer patients and their families. I am indebted to Dr. W. Scott McDougal's book, *Prostate Disease*, and to Mr. Dennis O'Hara for much of this information.

General Information

Prostate Cancer Support Network
1128 North Charles Street
Baltimore, MD 21201
800-828-7866

Prostate Health Council
American Foundation for Urologic Disease
1128 North Charles Street
Baltimore, MD 21201
800-242-2383

For general information about prostate cancer, and the address of the cancer support group nearest to you.

American Cancer Society
(chapters in all states, and most cities)
800-ACS-2345

Cancer Information Service
800-4-CANCER
For detailed information from the National Cancer Institute.

Support Groups
Us-Too
930 N. York Road, Suite 50
Hinsdale, IL 60521-2993
800-808-7866

Man-to-Man
Contact your local American Cancer Society for information.

Both of these are helpful, grass-roots organizations, and they usually meet at regular intervals of once or twice a month. Both welcome new members, and are an excellent source of information, counsel, sympathy, and experience.

Prostate Cancer On-Line
There is an ever-growing amount of information you can access on

the Web, if you are computer literate. It is expanding too fast to list every site, let alone the many on-line discussion groups. On the Internet, Usenet is worth reaching, particularly for information about new treatments, at <sci.med.prostate.cancer>.

World Wide Web pages that may be worth checking include:

<http://www.comed.com/prostate>
and
<http://oncolink.upenn.edu/disease/prostate/index.html>

However, there is so much information out there available to anybody who knows how to find it that it would be impossible to list it all here. Once again, your local American Cancer Society or support group will probably be able to help you separate the wheat from the chaff. Most support groups have at least one member who is an expert on the Internet and can advise you on where to find what you want to know without wasting your time or getting reams of medical information you don't need and can't interpret.

Remember: Your best resource is somebody who has had the disease and survived, and the best way of finding people like that is to join a support group.